The Super Aspirin Cure for Arthritis

Includes:

■ How the super aspirins can successfully treat osteoarthritis, rheumatoid arthritis, fibromyalgia, bursitis, tendinitis, carpal tunnel syndrome, and other joint-related diseases

■ What new treatments and drugs are on the horizon, including a possible arthritis vaccine and much more

■ The latest tests to diagnose and determine your specific type of arthritis

■ Five simple steps to pain-free living, including suggested exercises and dietary changes

The Super Aspirin Cure for Arthritis shows how, starting today, you can chart your path to a pain-free future.

D1359886

The Super Aspirin Cure for Arthritis

What You Need to Know About
the Breakthrough Drugs That
Stop Pain and Reverse Arthritis
Symptoms Without Side Effects

Harris H. McIlwain, M.D.
Debra Fulghum Bruce

🐓 **Bantam Books**

New York / Toronto / London / Sydney / Auckland

**The Super Aspirin Cure
for Arthritis**

PUBLISHING HISTORY
A Bantam Book / February 1999

ISBN 0-553-58107-4

PRINTED IN THE UNITED STATES OF AMERICA

OPM   10 9 8 7 6 5 4 3 2 1

To our mothers,

Cordelia Bryant McIlwain
and
Jewel Holden Fulghum

Acknowledgments

....

In our quest to give accurate and up-to-date
information on arthritis and the breakthrough
medications, we have received generous research
assistance from a very gifted group
of family, friends, and colleagues.

We express our gratitude to:
Allyn Gauthier; Ashley E. Bruce; Brittnye
Bruce; Claire Bruce; Hugh Cruse, M.P.H.;
Kimberly McIlwain; Laura McIlwain, M.D.;
Matthew Silliman; Michael McIlwain;
Robert G. Bruce III.

Note to Readers

....

The material in this book is for informational purposes only. It is not intended to serve as a diagnosis tool or prescription manual, or to replace the advice and care of your medical doctor. Although every effort has been made to provide the most up-to-date information, the medical science in this field and the information about Super Aspirins and other breakthrough medications are rapidly changing. Therefore, we strongly recommend that you consult with your doctor before attempting any of the treatments or programs discussed in this book. The authors and publisher expressly disclaim responsibility for any adverse effects that may result from the use or application of the information contained in this book.

To protect their privacy, pseudonyms have been used for the individual patients mentioned in this book.

Contents

Foreword

....

As an arthritis specialist for twenty-five years, who has treated thousands of patients, I wrote this book to share with you exciting information about the new Super Aspirins—the popular name for COX-2 inhibitors—and other breakthrough arthritis medications that are starting to come on the market and signal a revolution in arthritis treatment. Seeing the great results in years of clinical trials, I know that these new arthritis medications can dramatically reduce your pain and stiffness and help you to be active again.

Why do I think the new Super Aspirins are a ''cure'' for arthritis? Because I consider a cure to be a partial or perhaps complete relief of symptoms. Although medical researchers have yet to find an absolute cure or cause for most types of arthritis, the medications and other treatments I describe in this book will work in most cases to reduce or end your arthritis pain—*without side effects*.

Once you understand the type of arthritis you have, whether osteoarthritis (the wear-and-tear disease associated with aging joints) or rheumatoid (inflammatory) arthritis, you can work with your doctor to find the best new treatment available for you.

After you've read this book talk to your doctor about your arthritis aches and pains. Be sure to get the proper tests for an accurate diagnosis. Then follow my 5 Steps to Pain-Free Living, outlined in chapter 9, to halt pain and joint damage. These important steps include regular applications of moist heat, daily exercise, a nutritious diet, and avoidance of arthritis triggers.

In chapter 10 I explain an array of complementary treatments that can help you control pain and increase mobility, from ancient healing disciplines such as chi gong and tai chi to herbal therapies and healing foods. But all the treatments in the world won't help unless you make a strong commitment today to control your arthritis pain.

As you stop pain with the new Super Aspirins and other breakthrough treatments, you will feel younger, more energetic, and finally pain free because *you* are managing your arthritis—your arthritis is not managing you.

Good luck!

Harris McIlwain, M.D.

....

CHAPTER 1

Super Aspirins
Stop Your Pain!

If you need someone to help you with gardening, you might call Anna. This sixty-three-year-old retired English professor grows prize-winning Don Juan roses and brings them to my office for patients to enjoy. Although she is active now, Anna could hardly get out of a chair less than two years ago because of osteoarthritis pain and stiffness in her hips. In fact, walking caused her so much pain that her husband would bring her to my office in a wheelchair.

Anna tried ibuprofen and then another nonsteroid antiinflammatory drug (NSAID, pronounced ''en-SAYD''), the typical prescription for arthritis. Although these medications worked for a while, she finally had to quit taking them because of their side effect—stomach pain from a peptic ulcer. Anna also took cortisone injections to temporarily decrease the inflammation and pain, but within a few weeks the pain returned.

It was not until she signed up for a clinical trial for one of the new COX-2 inhibitors, popularly known as Super Aspirins, that she finally felt relief. After six weeks on the medication, Anna called my office in tears—but not because of the pain. These were tears of joy, because Anna could walk around the block with her three-year-old grandson—for the first time in his life.

Although we celebrate athletes' victories on the field, most of us are unaware of the pain athletes suffer when they finally throw in the towel. Jack, now retired from professional football where he played fullback for almost a decade, was thirty-two years old when I diagnosed him with osteoarthritis in the ankles and knees. Years of wear and tear, combined with old injuries to these joints, had caused them to erode, and Jack was in pain most of the time. For a while, he found some relief with traditional arthritis medications such as ibuprofen, but when he took the prescribed dosage, he felt nauseated and had stomach pains. Within a few months, I was treating Jack for arthritis and for gastrointestinal complaints.

When Jack said he couldn't even keep up with his five-year-old son at the beach because of arthritis pain, I realized that this young athlete felt sidelined from daily life. I suggested he participate in a clinical trial for the new Super Aspirins. He did, and this retired athlete went from being inactive to swimming daily at the local YMCA, riding a stationary bike for thirty minutes at a time, and taking long walks with his son. He felt so much better that five months later, he was hired to be the head coach for a local high school football team, and today he runs up and down the field, keeping up with his players.

Judith, thirty-four, lived with severe arthritis pain for three years. At first this active mother of two preschoolers ignored the increasing pain and stiffness in her hands and feet and took aspirin or ibuprofen to control it. Yet after a few months she found herself waking up an hour early each day to soak in a warm bath to decrease her pain and stiffness before driving her children to preschool. When she got home, Judith was exhausted from the drive and would nap until it was time to pick her children up at noon. When her knees and hips began to ache constantly, making it very difficult to sleep at night, much less care for her children, she began to worry. And when her younger daughter was ill one night and Judith could barely get out of bed without feeling intense pain, she knew she needed help.

Her primary care doctor diagnosed her with osteoarthritis. Yet after trying several different traditional NSAIDs, including ibuprofen and naproxen, Judith was experiencing even more swelling, pain, and fatigue than before and she had to hire help to care for her children. When I saw her for the first time, she was very distressed. Using some specific arthritis tests, including blood tests and x-rays, I discovered that she had rheumatoid arthritis. She volunteered to take part in a clinical trial of a new rheumatoid arthritis medication. After a few weeks, Judith reported almost completely alleviated joint pain, swelling, and stiffness. And she felt so reenergized that she resumed her normal activities, including caring for her two children by herself.

What Super Aspirins Can Do for You

As a board-certified rheumatologist and gerontologist, I've treated thousands of arthritis patients for the past twenty-five years. I'm part of the Tampa Medical Group; we have three large pain clinics on Florida's Gulf Coast and see hundreds of patients each week.

Because I diagnose and treat pain-related diseases daily, I am passionate about finding new treatment breakthroughs to help my patients ease the symptoms of their diseases. Arthritis today affects some 43 million Americans—one out of seven—including half of those over age sixty-five. And those numbers continue to grow.

Nearly everyone with arthritis takes aspirin or other NSAIDs to reduce inflammation and pain. Once the inflammation lessens, your pain also decreases, allowing for better mobility. But, as you may have experienced, although aspirin and traditional NSAIDs such as ibuprofen, naproxen, or ketoprofen give excellent pain relief, they also cause stomach problems and have a high risk of gastrointestinal complications, including bleeding ulcers. And the older you are, the more likely you'll experience unwanted side effects from aspirin and NSAIDs. With the number of Americans older than sixty-five rapidly increasing each year, the demand for a solution to inflammation and pain without side effects will only continue to skyrocket.

I have performed clinical trials with an array of experimental medications for more than two decades, hoping to identify those that give the best relief. I have found some drugs to be virtual lifesavers, while others have not been as helpful because of unwanted side effects.

For the past three years my colleagues and I at the Tampa Medical Group, along with other doctors nationwide, conducted clinical trials of a new class of drugs being developed for arthritis treatment: COX-2 inhibitors, popularly known as the Super Aspirins. Of course, anytime I've given a patient any treatment considered experimental, I'm always wondering what the negative side effect might be. Yet when the results of our clinical trials on the Super Aspirins were compared with trial conclusions from across the nation involving more than ten thousand adult men and women of all ages, the verdict was repeatedly the same. *In all the studies, researchers concluded that Super Aspirins control the pain and stiffness of osteoarthritis and rheumatoid arthritis but without peptic ulcers and bleeding, the side effects commonly associated with regular aspirin or with NSAIDs such as ibuprofen, naproxen, or ketoprofen.*

The breakthrough Super Aspirins that will be coming to the market as Celebrex, Vioxx, and Mobic have been proven in study after study to relieve the pain and stiffness associated with virtually all types of arthritis *with few side effects.* Super Aspirins are the cutting edge in arthritis treatment, the viable alternative for the thousands of arthritis sufferers who can't take traditional arthritis medications—aspirin and NSAIDs—because of their side effects of stomach upset or gastrointestinal problems. With the reduced risk of gastrointestinal side effects, Super Aspirins can be used at full doses, achieving a much greater anti-inflammatory- and pain-relieving effect. (Those who need the full NSAID effect are also those at the highest risk of unwanted and serious side effects.)

More Exciting Results and Uses

The first of the new generation of Super Aspirins is now being produced. Although these COX-2 inhibitors will be touted as pain relievers, scientists have also discovered that COX-2 is also involved in colon cancer, Alzheimer's disease, and other medical conditions. Is it possible that long-term use of Super Aspirins may protect or prevent colon cancer or Alzheimer's disease? The jury is still out, but the preliminary scientific evidence is extremely hopeful. I discuss those studies in more detail in chapter 7.

How Super Aspirins Work

How do the Super Aspirins do what aspirin and NSAIDs do but without side effects? Here's a summary of the crucial difference, which I describe in more detail in chapters 6 and 7.

Aspirin and traditional NSAIDs work by blocking the body's production of prostaglandins—the chemicals that cause inflammation, pain, swelling, and, in some types of arthritis, even joint destruction. In 1971 British researcher John Vane demonstrated in Nobel Prize–winning studies that aspirin inhibits the functioning of *cyclooxygenase,* or COX, an enzyme that cells need to make prostaglandins.

It's the pain caused by prostaglandins that bothers most of us; the prostaglandins send messages to cells that trigger inflammation. Aspirin and traditional NSAIDs block the prostaglandin, thus blocking inflammation and reducing pain and stiffness. But prostaglandins send a few good messages as well, protecting the stomach lining and kidneys. So by blocking prostaglandins entirely, aspirin and traditional

NSAIDs leave you vulnerable to the risk of stomach ulcers, bleeding, and even kidney damage.

In the early 1990s scientists discovered that there were actually two forms of the COX enzyme. They realized that the COX-1 enzyme was very common in normal tissues and helped maintain their normal functioning in the stomach, kidney, and other areas, while the COX-2 form controlled inflammation, mainly in joints. So, as scientists realized in this breakthrough discovery, the real culprit in inflammation and pain is the COX-2 enzyme.

Until now, all of the traditional NSAIDs on the market, such as aspirin and ibuprofen, block both COX-2 *and* COX-1. Although stopping COX-2 reduces inflammation, blocking COX-1 leaves many vulnerable to serious side effects involving the stomach and kidneys. Some may block COX-1 or COX-2 more than others. You need pain relief from arthritis, but it must be safe.

Successful Clinical Trials with Remarkable Results

In nationwide clinical trials involving more than ten thousand men and women of all ages, researchers have concluded that Super Aspirins control the pain and stiffness of osteoarthritis and rheumatoid arthritis without the side effects commonly associated with aspirin or NSAIDs, such as gastrointestinal distress. The clinical studies also included surveys that measured the drugs' effects on patients' overall quality of life. Across the board, patients felt better physically, so it was much easier for them to walk, climb stairs, or carry groceries, activities of daily living we take for granted. It is not surprising to any arthritis patient that if pain is relieved, they feel better all over!

Throughout the Super Aspirins' trials in our clinics, many of our patients received the same great benefits—a dramatic decrease in arthritis pain with no side effects. Patients shared with me stories of the miraculous pain relief they experienced taking Celebrex, Vioxx or Mobic—the brand names of the new Super Aspirins.

Here's an overview of some of the exciting results; more detailed study results appear in chapter 7.

■ In studies involving 1,000 patients with osteoarthritis, researchers found that Celebrex relieved as much pain as naproxen, a standard traditional NSAID used for treatment of osteoarthritis—but without the serious gastrointestinal side effects associated with naproxen.

Rita, sixty-seven, with osteoarthritis in the knees, said, "I knew that if I lost weight, my arthritis pain would improve. Yet how could I exercise or be active when my knees hurt too much to even walk? After starting on Celebrex, the pain virtually diminished, and I started a regular walking program with some friends. Now I walk two miles a day without any pain at all and am finally losing weight. It has changed my life."

■ Clinical trials on 1,100 rheumatoid arthritis patients revealed that those who received Celebrex experienced reduced pain and swelling in their joints, as did those who received naproxen. The difference is that while NSAIDs such as naproxen are effective medicines in some cases of rheumatoid arthritis, they may cause side effects such as stomach upset.

■ Super Aspirin clinical trials with osteoarthritis patients involving the new medication Vioxx showed that Vioxx is as effective as many other traditional NSAIDs but with less indigestion, nausea, peptic ulcers, and intestinal bleeding.

Candace, forty-one, with osteoarthritis in the ankles, said, "After dancing professionally for nearly two decades, my ankles are fifty years older than the rest of my body. Before taking Vioxx, I could only wear sturdy tennis shoes, even for evening wear, because of the tremendous pain and stiffness. Now I'm able to dress like a normal person. The pain has greatly diminished and I feel lucky to be active and have a life again.''

■ Some large Super Aspirin studies conducted in Europe of more than twenty thousand patients with osteoarthritis included treatment with Mobic, diclofenac (Voltaren), and piroxicam (Feldene). Just as with all the Super Aspirin research, these results on the Mobic studies confirmed the relief of arthritis pain, but with fewer cases of indigestion, nausea, abdominal pain, and peptic ulcers.

Ron, forty-four, with osteoarthritis in the knees and back, said, ''I was in a Mobic trial for osteoarthritis. While the new medicine was not intended for my severe lower back pain, I found excellent relief for both types of arthritis pain. I even went bowling a few weeks ago with some friends.''

Super Aspirins Help All Types of Pain

Although the Super Aspirin clinical trials focused on specific pain, such as osteoarthritis in the knee or hip, or rheumatoid arthritis, patients of all ages and with all types of pain found amazing relief with these new medications. Celebrex, Vioxx, and Mobic seemed to relieve pain associated with fibromyalgia, menstrual cramps, carpal tunnel, bursitis, golfer's and tennis elbow, and tendinitis.

■ Emily, thirty-three, with rheumatoid arthritis, found that Celebrex relieved her joint pain enough for her to enjoy a tai chi class in her neighborhood, and that it also helped with menstrual pain, relief that not even ibuprofen could give.

■ Mac, forty-four, with osteoarthritis in the knee and carpal tunnel in his right wrist from overuse on the computer, participated in the Vioxx study and found relief for the arthritis and repetitive stress injury.

■ Bob, forty-six, with osteoarthritis in the knee from an old track injury and a chronic case of "golfer's elbow," signed up for the Mobic study and found that this Super Aspirin ended both problems—no more pain in either joint.

No Side Effects

Super Aspirins give amazing arthritis pain relief without stomach discomfort. The most common side effects of Super Aspirins reported so far are diarrhea and headache, but keep in mind that these side effects also occurred in *placebo* patients, those patients who were given an "inactive" medication. Nonetheless, the side effects were not severe enough to make patients stop taking the medication. A word of caution: as with any medication, not everyone who takes the Super Aspirins responds with reduced pain. Your doctor should help you decide if one of these medications would be worthwhile to try.

More Breakthrough Drugs
for Rheumatoid Arthritis

Our patients also participated in clinical trials on new drugs for rheumatoid arthritis, a serious type of arthritis, which I describe in chapter 8. These and other breakthrough medicines offer dramatic improvement in severe rheumatoid arthritis without the side effects of the older medicines on the stomach, liver, and kidney. If you have rheumatoid arthritis, excellent new medications are available that let you control the pain and stiffness and actually alter the course of your disease, reducing it from something terrible to something that may be inconvenient but manageable.

Some of these new medications, such as Enbrel and Arava, have received FDA approval; others will be reviewed in the next year by the FDA, and as they become available, they will transform the way we treat arthritis pain and inflammation.

The reactions of those who took other breakthrough medications in clinical trials for more serious forms of rheumatoid arthritis or inflammatory types of arthritis were just as encouraging:

- Anthony, thirty-eight, with rheumatoid arthritis, said, "After the Arava, I can get up and go to work without feeling like my body has given up on me. After working a full day, I can now play ball with my son. I thought I would never be able to do that again."

- Kim, twenty-six, with rheumatoid arthritis, said, "I was lucky to start on Arava before there were signs of joint damage. The pain I once felt has diminished by eighty percent. I now hope that being more active will help me get strong enough to fight this disease."

- Ginny, forty-six, with rheumatoid arthritis, said, "Enbrel gave me my life back! I even went to the beach with my teenagers and their friends for a week this summer and was able to enjoy it completely."

Will These Medications Help You?

By now you may be wondering if Super Aspirins or other breakthrough medications will help your arthritis pain. There is only one sure way to find out: ask your doctor about these new medications, and see which ones are now available to treat arthritis pain. Although some of these medications are already on the market, others are in the final stages of clinical trials and are not yet available.

I know that you, too, can shut *off* pain with the Super Aspirins. However, the earlier you begin proper treatment— treatment aimed at your specific arthritis problem—the better the results will be. Working with your doctor, make it your goal to become an expert on your own arthritis. Chapter 2 is an arthritis primer, and in subsequent chapters you can learn about the signs and symptoms of the main types of arthritis: chapter 3 covers osteoarthritis and other wear-and-tear arthritis types, as well as fibromyalgia; chapter 4 covers inflammatory types of arthritis, including rheumatoid arthritis. It's crucial to have an accurate diagnosis of your arthritis, and in chapter 5 I describe the various diagnostic tests available.

Your goal should be to render your arthritis—whether mild, moderate, or severe—a controlled condition in which you can get around and do the activities you wish—without pain or stiffness. And that starts with medication. I explain what's wrong with traditional arthritis medicine in chapter 6 and then discuss the Super Aspirins in chapter 7 and other breakthrough medications in chapter 8.

But in conjunction with medicine, you need to take five more steps for pain-free living. In chapter 9, I outline the program I prescribe for all my patients—along with their medication. Optimal pain control requires regular exercise, along with other measures such as moist heat and a healthful diet. In my practice, I spend much time convincing patients that exercise is critical. The chances of your joints becoming limber and muscles getting stronger greatly increase with exercise. And by eating certain foods high in omega-3 fatty acids, such as fish, or eliminating foods that are known "arthritis triggers," you can gain more pain control. There are also a host of complementary treatments, described in chapter 10, that help ease arthritis pain. When surgery is necessary, your options are outlined in chapter 11.

Who has time for arthritis pain, much less serious gastrointestinal problems caused by medications? Certainly not me or you or millions of other arthritis sufferers. So by learning about the breakthrough medications available and complementary steps to ease your pain, let's make your arthritis something that you can manage.

....

CHAPTER 2

Arthritis 101

To understand how the new Super Aspirins and other medicines will literally shut *off* your pain, you need to first understand what switches *on* arthritis pain. *Arthritis* actually means "inflammation in or around the joints"—and this inflammation in your body causes the pain, swelling, and stiffness you feel.

For some people, such as my patient Wendy, arthritis develops gradually over a period of months or years. This young attorney was studying for the bar exam when she first noticed pain and stiffness in her hands and shoulders. Thinking it stemmed from the lack of physical activity inherent in the long hours of reading and writing in preparation for the exam, Wendy took aspirin several times a day and made a personal commitment to exercise more after the test. It wasn't until several days after the bar exam, when she could not get out of bed because of severe pain in her knees and ankles, that she knew her condition was more serious. This pain was unlike any she had ever experienced, with both knees swollen to almost twice their normal size and the skin reddened and warm to the touch. When she tried to walk to the bathroom, she could hardly put weight on her feet without feeling a crushing pain in both knees and ankles. Wendy was just twenty-four years old when I diagnosed her with rheumatoid arthritis, a serious type of inflammatory arthritis that needs immediate attention to prevent joint damage.

Other people may go to bed feeling no pain at all, then awake with painful, inflamed, or swollen joints or with deep muscle pain. Sometimes the joints feel warm to the touch. Keep in mind that although sore or painful muscles and joints can result from yard work, weekend sports, or other activities, these types of minor aches and pains usually go away after a few days. When the pain, stiffness, or swelling lasts longer than a few days or returns again and again, it could be a warning sign of the more persistent problem of arthritis.

No matter how their arthritis feels or what type they may have, the number of people suffering with arthritis is astounding and will only escalate as baby boomers enter their fifties and sixties. According to the Centers for Disease Control (CDC) and the Arthritis Foundation, in 1960 nearly 28.5 million people in the United States had arthritis. In 1990, more than 37.9 million Americans had some form of arthritis, and by 1995, 40 million Americans (one in six people) had some form of arthritis. Arthritis currently affects more

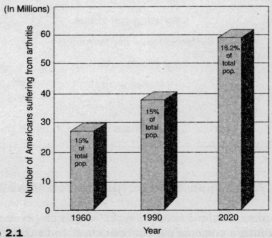

Figure 2.1

than 43 million people, and the CDC projects that by the year 2020 more than 59.4 million Americans—almost 20 percent of the entire population—will suffer from arthritis (Figure 2.1).

THE MOST COMMON TYPES OF ARTHRITIS

· ·

OSTEOARTHRITIS TYPES

Osteoarthritis

Fibromyalgia

Bursitis

Tendinitis

Carpal tunnel syndrome

INFLAMMATORY ARTHRITIS

Rheumatoid arthritis

Ankylosing spondylitis

Systemic lupus erythematosus

Gout (Gouty arthritis)

Pseudogout

PMR (polymyalgia rheumatica)

Others

What Type of Arthritis Do You Have?

With more than one hundred types of arthritis, even experienced arthritis specialists can have trouble deciding which type of arthritis you have. Yet the idea that all arthritis is alike has led sufferers to try treatments that have little effect on their particular symptoms. What works for someone else's arthritis may not work for you. Because each type of arthritis may need a different type of treatment, an accurate diagnosis is crucial. Once you know what causes the pain, you can take steps to relieve it properly and continue to be active.

It makes it easier if we divide arthritis into two main categories: osteoarthritis and inflammatory arthritis. Osteoarthritis, or degenerative arthritis, includes the wear-and-tear arthritis types, while the inflammatory types of arthritis are those in which the linings of joints become inflamed.

Signs and Symptoms

Arthritis can attack almost any of the body's joints and commonly hits the hands, wrists, elbows, shoulders, knees, ankles, feet, neck, or back. It can even attack the jaw. Some patients say they found joints they didn't even know they had!

Some types of arthritis attack a regular pattern of joints. For example, osteoarthritis frequently affects joints that bear weight over the years, such as the knees, hips, or lower back. Rheumatoid arthritis usually affects the hands, wrists, elbows, shoulders, knees, ankles, and feet in some combination. Gout is famous for attacking the big toe.

Just as there is a usual pattern of attack, most people affected by arthritis report a regular pattern of symptoms, particularly pain and stiffness, when they first get up in the morning. You may notice that it takes a few minutes to "loosen up"—or many hours. One middle-aged woman with rheumatoid arthritis said it took her "twice as long to feel half as good" as she used to feel.

But once you get up and move around to alleviate the stiffness, you may feel stiff again if you sit for more than a few minutes at a time. Most arthritis sufferers will admit to pain and stiffness after sitting in a class, in church, at a theater, in a car, or while working at the computer. In these situations, it may take them a few minutes to get going again.

"They think I'm lazy," fifty-two-year-old Ginah told me, referring to her co-workers. "I tell them I have arthritis, but they think it's my excuse." I tell all my patients that it is common to feel tired with arthritis, even too tired to finish daily activities that were once easy. In fact, for millions of men and women, the fatigue can be even more bothersome than the joint pain.

As Ginah experienced, this never-ending fatigue is often a great source of stress and misunderstanding among friends and family, who think the arthritis sufferer is lazy. A good response to skeptics might be to ask them about the last time they had the flu. Ask them to remember the achiness, stiffness, and unending fatigue they experienced, then imagine these feelings lasting all day, every day of their lives. That is how arthritis feels.

Other problems can come with arthritis, too. Besides pain, stiffness, swelling, and fatigue, you may have fever, lose weight, and get rashes on your skin. Internal organ disease may coincide with arthritis and affect the kidney, heart, and other internal organs. Because there are many causes of fever, weight loss, or skin rashes, it's important to talk to your doctor to be sure no other problems are present.

If you have any of the signs of arthritis symptoms on page 17 with arthritis, talk to your doctor about the new treatments.

Not only does arthritis cause physical pain, it results in 39 million doctor visits each year and is second only to heart disease as a cause of work disability. Combined with costly treatments, the loss of work is devastating to patients and their families and can drain retirement savings. Experts estimate the total cost of arthritis in the United States rose from $21 billion in 1980 to $149 billion in 1992. With the increase in the number of people age fifty-five and older, the number with arthritis will only skyrocket, driving the cost up as well. Severe arthritis can lower earnings by 25 to 50 percent in those who continue to work.

COMMON SIGNS AND SYMPTOMS OF ARTHRITIS

....

Stiffness in the morning on arising

Weight loss

Fever

Rash

Discoloration of the fingers when cold

Sensitivity to the sun

Painful urination

Genital ulcers

Eye inflammation

Sinusitis

Abdominal pain

Diarrhea

Fatigue

Shortness of breath

Difficulty swallowing

Headache

Hypertension

Loss of hair

Mouth ulcers

Back pain

Vision changes

Eye dryness

Chest pain

The ongoing stress of arthritis combined with medical bills, loss of work, and worry about the future can contribute to depression and other emotional reactions that further limit your ability to deal effectively with daily living. Many with arthritis feel constant pain that causes stiffness and immobility. The inability to exercise and remain active can also lead to feelings of depression that add to your lethargy and fatigue. When you don't move around, the chances are great that your pain, stiffness, and anxiety will increase even more.

Understanding Leads to Relief

When I diagnose patients with arthritis, much of their anxiety and distress stems from a lack of knowledge about the disease. Not only are they frightened because they hurt and have difficulty moving the arthritic limb or joint, but their uneasiness about living with a chronic illness is overwhelming. Education helps them overcome these fears.

Using the information in the next two chapters, you can better understand the type of arthritis you may have. Then, along with a Super Aspirin or other medication and the 5 Steps to Pain-Free Living (chapter 9), you will be better equipped to control your arthritis.

....

CHAPTER 3

Osteoarthritis, Fibromyalgia, and Other Wear-and-Tear Problems

If you've ever had painful joints after a weekend of activities, you know how difficult it can be to get out of bed. Margie, a former college basketball player, is familiar with this pain and, more recently, with the pain of arthritis. "Osteoarthritis? I am forty-one and living proof that you don't have to be old to feel the effects of this ailment," she said. "Not only do my joints ache in the morning, but after doing yard work or spending a day cleaning our home, I have to soak in our Jacuzzi for relief."

Margie's story is one you might relate to: an athlete as a young adult, a sedentary career, a weight gain of twenty pounds since college, and now inactive because her knees and hips hurt "all day, every day." While she believes in exercise to maintain good health, Margie cannot remember the last time she really tried to get back in shape and added, "When I exercise, my knees hurt so badly, I immediately stop. Why do I want to inflict more pain on what I already live with?"

The good news is that Margie found help with Celebrex, one of the Super Aspirins. She volunteered for a Super Aspirins clinical trial for osteoarthritis patients and in less than a month felt such relief from pain and stiffness that she was out walking the track at a nearby high school. Today she has lost the extra weight and feels in charge of her life again. She is able to be as active as she wants and enjoys swimming and biking with her children after school.

Osteoarthritis and other wear-and-tear types of arthritis do hurt—if left untreated. Now, with one of the Super Aspirins, along with regular applications of moist heat and an ongoing exercise program, almost anyone can move beyond the pain.

Osteoarthritis

Osteoarthritis (OA), or "wear and tear" arthritis, is the most common type of arthritis. OA is more common in adults over fifty, and it affects an estimated 85 percent of the population age seventy and older. More than 20 million Americans suffer from OA. Although women account for about 65 percent of all arthritis cases, they account for 74 percent of osteoarthritis cases (15.3 million women). It is most common in joints required to bear weight over the years, such as the knees, hips, feet, and spine and often develops gradually over months or years (figure 3.2). Except for the intense pain in the affected joint, one usually does not feel sick, and there is no unusual fatigue, as with other types of arthritis.

Age-related wear and tear and injuries may cause minor damage to the cartilage that will never be completely repaired. The injury might be major and obvious, like a knee injury in sports, when cartilage is damaged, or minor injuries can accumulate over the years and ultimately damage the cartilage, leading to osteoarthritis. Gradually, as more and more damage occurs, the cartilage begins to wear away or doesn't work as well to cushion the joint. For example, extra stress on knees from excess weight or obesity can further damage knee cartilage, allowing it to wear out faster than normal. (Interestingly, the hands also seem to be at higher risk for osteoarthritis when a person is overweight.) As the cartilage cushioning the joint becomes worn, its smoothness is lost, which can cause pain when the joint moves. Along

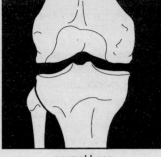

normal knee   osteoarthritis

Figure 3.1 A normal knee joint compared to
osteoarthritis in the knee.

with the pain, you may hear a grating sound when the roughened cartilage on the surface of the bones rubs together. Bumps may appear, especially on the fingers and feet.

Who's at Risk?

Although age, overuse, and being overweight are big risk factors, OA can also occur in younger, otherwise fit adults, especially after an injury. The weekend athlete who injures a knee or an ankle playing tennis or softball may develop osteoarthritis in the injured joint. Those who enjoy dancing or running could develop osteoarthritis in their ankles in their thirties or forties. Someone who has fallen and injured her back is also a prime candidate for osteoarthritis in the lower spine.

RISK FACTORS FOR OSTEOARTHRITIS
....

Age (older than forty-five years)

Injury

Heavy, constant joint use

Athletics (wear and tear and injuries from athletics)

Overweight

Knee surgery

Abnormal joint positions

Changing forces (putting weight on one knee or hip)

Joint injury from other types of arthritis

Gender (between forty-five and fifty-five, the chance of developing OA is the same for men and women; after age fifty-five, OA is more common in women)

Lack of exercise (weak muscles giving no support to aging joints)

What You May Feel

"I thought arthritis was something I'd get when I retired," says Shannon, one of my younger osteoarthritis patients, who was diagnosed with OA in her hands at thirty-one. Many times we see young women in their thirties like Shannon develop arthritis in their hands, even without much wear-and-tear damage, and it commonly runs in families. This type of arthritis may limit itself mainly to the hands, usually affecting the joints nearest the fingernails and at the base of the thumb. (Figure 3.3)

You may first notice signs of osteoarthritis in your feet, which may hurt frequently because osteoarthritis causes bones to become enlarged. This creates added pressure against the shoe, a nearby bone, or the ground. The body reacts by forming a corn or callus, a deformity that can actually change the shape of the foot. Sometimes more corns and calluses are caused by the misshapen foot and poorly fitting shoes. This is especially common after age forty or

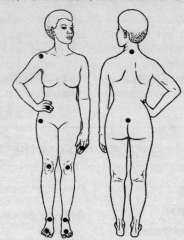

Figure 3.2

fifty. Your doctor may recommend a custom-made shoe or surgery to correct the problem.

In OA the patient usually feels well except for the affected joint. Osteoarthritis causes no internal organ problems. You may feel stiff for a few minutes on arising in the morning,

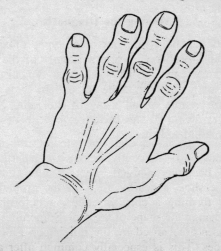

Figure 3.3

and you may feel some stiffness after sitting for a short period of time, but these symptoms are usually not as severe as in patients with inflammatory types of arthritis. You may feel pain and swelling in your joints, which may make it hard to walk or to arise from a chair due to knee, hip, or back pain. Opening jars or writing may be painful when the hands are affected.

SYMPTOMS OF OSTEOARTHRITIS

....

Deep, aching pain in joint	Pain when walking
Swelling of joint	Difficulty gripping objects
Joint warm to the touch	Difficulty dressing or combing hair
Morning stiffness	
Stiffness after resting	Difficulty sitting or bending over
Fatigue	

Making the Diagnosis

Blood tests can help rule out other types of arthritis and other medical problems, while a sample of the joint fluid from the knee can also show changes typical of osteoarthritis. Usually by the time a patient gets treatment, changes are visible on an x-ray of the joint. X-rays may reveal a narrowing of the cartilage, but no destruction as with rheumatoid arthritis.

Fibromyalgia

Fibromyalgia syndrome (FMS) is a complex arthritis-type disorder characterized by widespread pain, decreased pain threshold or tender points, and incapacitating fatigue. It affects 10 million Americans. Although there is no specific laboratory test or abnormal x-ray finding to diagnose FMS, the symptoms of the disease are very real and can be successfully treated *once a proper diagnosis is made*. However, fibromyalgia is not usually diagnosed very early. In some studies patients suffered from pain and fatigue for three to four years before being diagnosed with fibromyalgia.

The cause of fibromyalgia is not known, but comprehensive studies in the past five years conclude that it may start after a serious illness or injury or other severe stress. It may represent a problem in the way the body manages pain signals so that pain is felt more easily and becomes prominent.

A study from the American College of Rheumatology suggests that fibromyalgia and chronic fatigue syndrome (CFS) may actually be the same disease, because fatigue is also severe in fibromyalgia, and symptoms seem to increase after periods of high stress or physical exertion, as with CFS.

Who's at Risk?

Fibromyalgia has been tagged a woman's disease because women are ten times as likely to get this disease as are men. The onset usually occurs between the ages of forty and fifty. Some patients develop fibromyalgia after an accident or after surgery.

What You May Feel

April came to our clinic complaining of searing pain in her back, neck, arms, and legs, along with throbbing headaches. She was stiff when she awoke in the mornings and felt continuously exhausted, which she described as flulike symptoms. She had not slept well in months, and the more tired she became, the more difficulty she had getting sound sleep. April also had abdominal cramps and diarrhea followed by bouts of constipation. She had specific tender "trigger" points on her back, shoulders, and hips, and no medicines had relieved these chronic symptoms.

FMS will cause the severe constant pain that April described. The deep, aching pain can be everywhere—the back, the neck, the arms and legs—and felt in the muscles and tendons around the joints. You may also have tender spots on your arms, legs, neck, and back, which are painful when touched or pressed with a finger. The locations of the tender points are not random but occur in predictable places (Figure 3.4).

POSSIBLE CONTRIBUTING CAUSES OF FIBROMYALGIA

....

Decrease in serotonin (a chemical in the body often associated with calming and anti-anxiety)

Aging

Female gender

High sensitivity to pain (even from normally nonpainful stimulation)

Inherited tendency

Magnesium deficiency

Menopause

Poor physical conditioning

Depression

Injury or accident

Flu

Sleep disorder

Stress

Surgery

Trauma to the nervous system

Fibromyalgia also causes severe fatigue that is always present, even after rest, and limits daily activities. It may feel more like exhaustion than sleepiness. Those with FMS may also have an inability to concentrate, or what they tag "fibro fog," making it difficult to focus at work.

Sleep is often interrupted by pain and is hard to improve, even with sleep medications. The lack of sleep can be frustrating, of course, and this alone can increase your fatigue.

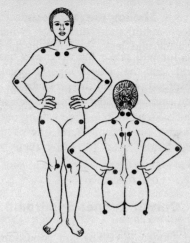

Figure 3.4

You may also have stiffness in the muscles and joints on arising, which may take hours to loosen up.

COMMON SYMPTOMS OF FIBROMYALGIA

Pain

Fatigue

Morning stiffness

Trigger points

Sleep problems

Anxiety

Difficulty concentrating

Depression

Swelling, numbness, and tingling in hands, arms, feet, and legs

Chronic headaches

Dryness in mouth, nose, or eyes

Restless legs syndrome

Irritable bowel syndrome

Urinary symptoms

Painful menstrual cramps

Discoloration of hands and feet (Raynaud's phenomenon) on cold exposure

Making the Diagnosis

Because FMS cannot be detected through x-rays or blood tests, your doctor will make the diagnosis based on overall clinical findings and the criteria for fibromyalgia, including chronic, widespread pain and the presence of at least eleven of the eighteen standard tender points (diagram on page 27). Along with the 5 Steps to Pain-Free Living outlined in chapter 9, your doctor may recommend one of the new Super Aspirins, successfully used for other types of arthritis in clinical trials.

Carpal Tunnel Syndrome

Carpal tunnel syndrome (CTS) is a condition in which the median nerve, which travels down the arm into the hand, becomes compressed as it passes through the bones in the wrist that form the carpal tunnel. Overuse can cause the tissues in the area to swell, and this swelling causes pressure on the median nerve.

Who's at Risk?

CTS can occur at any age but occurs more frequently without cause in those age fifty and up. It affects two million Americans at a cost to business of $20 billion annually, and is reported 1.7 times more often by working women than by men. More women than men also experience musculoskeletal injuries to the hand, wrist, arm, and shoulder caused by child care responsibilities requiring lifting and bending. Younger people usually get CTS as a result of an injury or repetitive stress on the wrist. Although CTS can happen to anyone, the following occupations and activities carry a greater risk:

- construction worker
- musician
- seamstress
- knitting

- typing
- hairdresser
- computer operator

Swelling in the hands caused by diabetes or pregnancy may also trigger CTS. Having rheumatoid arthritis places you at higher risk of CTS as well.

What You May Feel

CTS symptoms include pain, tingling, or numbness in the thumb and next three fingers, but not in the little finger. You may also feel swelling in your fingers. Sometimes the pain travels from the hand to the elbow.

The pain, numbness, and tingling usually worsen at night and while driving or holding the telephone. Some claim the symptoms increase when the hand is warm and decrease when it is cool. You may even wake up with one or both hands asleep and have to shake them to regain feeling.

As CTS progresses, your hand may become noticeably weaker so that opening a jar or grasping a hairbrush may become difficult. You may drop items easily and think you're just plain clumsy when, in fact, the CTS has weakened your grip.

Making the Diagnosis

Your doctor can diagnose CTS after a complete physical examination and review of your medical history. He will notice the type of pain you have and the specific places on your hand that it occurs. Tests, including an electrical nerve conduction test, may be helpful in obtaining an accurate diagnosis. X-rays and blood tests are usually performed. Depending on the exact cause, treatment may include one of the Super Aspirins, along with a splint for your wrist, a local injection of cortisone to reduce the swelling around the nerve, or possibly a minor outpatient surgical procedure.

Bursitis

Bursitis is inflammation of one of the sacs around tendons or muscles that allow them to move smoothly. With bursitis, you will feel severe pain anytime your muscles or tendons move, when there is movement of the affected joint, or even when there is pressure on the joint. The pain can be mild or severe and may last for days, weeks, or months and can occur around the shoulders, hips, knees, elbows, or buttocks. Repetitive movements, such as throwing, painting, or yard work, especially if not done regularly, can frequently trigger an attack of bursitis. For example, bursitis in the shoulder can happen after overdoing weekend activities around the house. This can make it very painful just to lift your arm above your shoulder.

There are many different causes of bursitis, but the most common is wear-and-tear changes and repetitive movements of the muscles and tendons as they slide through the bursa sac. An injury can also cause inflammation of the area and pain on movement. Your doctor can make sure there are no other causes present, such as infection, which require specific treatment. If it is just bursitis, one of the new Super Aspirins may be prescribed along with moist heat and rest, followed by gradually increasing exercise.

Tendinitis

Tendinitis is inflammation of one of the tendons that attaches a muscle to a bone. This can cause severe pain, especially when the muscle is used. One of the most common types of tendinitis occurs at the elbow, where it is called tennis elbow because the movements in tennis can trigger an attack. Other common sites are the shoulder, elbow, Achilles tendon, or the heel.

Tendinitis can happen alone or along with true arthritis in the nearby joint. In some cases, tendinitis can progress to what we call a frozen shoulder, when the ligaments and tendons around the shoulder progressively stiffen until the joint can barely move without pain. Super Aspirins, along with the 5-step treatment plan, can help ease your tendinitis and give you pain-free mobility again.

Trigger Finger

Trigger finger is a common cause of hand pain. It is due to inflammation of a sheath around a tendon that moves the finger. This is usually caused by wear-and-tear changes, and either the tendon swells or the sheath around the tendon shrinks. The tendon slides less easily in one direction than the other, which causes the pain and makes the finger snap or catch like a trigger when it moves. The finger may stop in a bent or in a straight position, and it may be painful to move it further. Patients feel the need to use their other hand to straighten or bend the trigger finger.

Usually, the more the trigger finger is used, the more painful it becomes. The trigger finger may improve when rested but usually requires an injection of cortisone to improve the inflammation around the tendon. If the injection does not work or does not last long enough, an outpatient surgery can fix the trigger-finger tendon problem.

Back Pain and Arthritis

Osteoarthritis is a common cause of back pain, which may be either sharp or dull and aching. This type of back pain can develop years after an injury because joints that are injured have a higher chance of developing arthritis later. The pain may start slowly, then increase over the years, as the spine's cartilage becomes more worn. You may notice stiffness when you awaken in the morning or after sitting for more than a few minutes.

But the exact causes of back pain are often not known. It can be called acute lower back (lumbar) strain, but the cause

of the strain may be an injury or may not be apparent at all.
At times there may be pressure on a nerve in the lower back.
Specific medical problems, including arthritis, fracture of
one of the bones in the spine because of osteoporosis (thinning of the bones), infections in the spine, internal organ
disease, and cancer, can cause acute back pain and are important to find. Acute back pain can be caused by lifting too
much weight at one time, but sometimes the pain occurs
when there is no lifting at all—just bending over. One patient
told us that the pain could come on if he leaned over to pick
up a feather!

Lumbar Stenosis

Osteoarthritis in the lumbar spine can lead to other causes of
back pain. It may cause a narrowing of the space that contains the nerve roots coming away from the spinal cord, putting pressure on the nerves, which results in lower back pain,
especially after walking a short distance. The pain can travel
down both legs and may stop after you rest for a few minutes.
As the condition worsens, the distance you can walk before
the severe pain begins gets shorter and shorter.

After diagnosis by your doctor, lumbar stenosis can be
treated with moist heat, exercise, and medications, such as
one of the Super Aspirins. If there is no improvement, injections of cortisone might give temporary relief or surgery may
be necessary to relieve the pressure on the nerves.

Ruptured Disc

Ruptured (herniated or slipped) disc usually can cause severe
back pain. The disc material and inflammation cause pressure on a nerve as it leaves the spine. The pain may worsen if
you cough or sneeze, and you may also feel pain, numbness
or tingling traveling down one leg (sciatica). Treatment for a
ruptured disc includes rest, moist heat to the back, and gradually increasing exercise. Medications such as a Super Aspirin
or traditional NSAID can help both the pain and inflamma-

tion. About 90 percent of cases do *not* need surgery, but if your symptoms continue without relief, surgery to remove the ruptured disc can give effective relief.

SELF-TEST FOR RUPTURED DISC

If you're experiencing back pain with pain down your leg, try the following self-test to see if you possibly have a ruptured disc: Lie flat on your bed, then raise your affected leg at the hip without bending your knee. Normally, you can probably lift this leg straight up at a 90-degree angle without pain. If you have pain in your back while doing this leg raise, *you may have a ruptured disc.* If there is numbness or tingling in the leg or foot, it could be a sign of nerve irritation. See your doctor for further advice.

Combined Causes of Back Pain

It is very common to have a combination of these causes of back pain. For example, osteoarthritis may be present, but trigger-point tenderness associated with fibromyalgia may make the pain much worse. It's important to determine this "combination" of causes to find the best way to treat your pain.

Remember that there are causes of back pain unrelated to osteoarthritis. Some internal organ problems can make pain travel to the back. Also, back pain can be caused by peptic ulcer disease ("stomach" ulcer), gallstones, and osteo-porosis-induced bone fractures in your back. Back pain can also be a symptom of an enlarged aorta (aortic aneurysm), some forms of cancer, and kidney problems. Each of these needs proper diagnosis and treatment, so check with your doctor to be sure no other causes of back pain are present.

With the new Super Aspirins, good treatment will be available for osteoarthritis, fibromyalgia, and other types of wear-and-tear problems outlined in this chapter. To get the best relief now and in the future, start early with a diagnosis and treatment. If you are still hesitant about using medications, some of the complementary treatments in chapter 10 such as bodyworks, chiropractic, or acupuncture may be your ticket to living pain free without drugs. If medications are needed, try acetaminophen or an over-the-counter NSAID. If you still have no relief, talk to your doctor. See if one of the Super Aspirins may help you control your pain without unwanted side effects.

....

CHAPTER 4

Rheumatoid Arthritis, Gout, and Other Inflammatory Types of Arthritis

"I moved my blanket and pillow to the living room couch so I wouldn't have to climb the stairs to our bedroom." Jack, 42

"I can't hold a cup of coffee in the morning because my joints ache so badly, so I sip it through a straw." Maryanne, 39

"Even though I don't have to be at work until nine A.M., I awaken at five A.M. just to loosen up my stiff joints so I don't hurt all day." Peter, 38

"My baby doesn't know what it's like to be rocked by her own mother. It hurts too much to hold her in my arms." Claire, 27

These were common statements made by patients with rheumatoid arthritis before Super Aspirins and other new arthritis medications.

Although osteoarthritis stems from the wear and tear of joints, the inflammatory types of arthritis such as rheumatoid arthritis occur when your immune system goes haywire and attacks the linings of the joints. Almost any joint can be involved, and the causes are known in only a few types.

With the inflammatory types of arthritis, you may feel pain, swelling, stiffness, and warmth around the joints, but this is even more limiting and severe than with osteoarthritis. Why? Because the prostaglandins that cause inflammation trigger enzymes that cause pain and swelling and also trigger other enzymes that attack the cartilage and bones in the joints. As your own immune cells and their products eat away at your cartilage, your bones will eventually erode. The areas of bones that become damaged and destroyed may be small, but over a few years, these changes can add up to joint deformity and limited use.

Treatments, including the Super Aspirins and traditional NSAIDs, try to block the enzymes, helping to improve the pain and swelling. The breakthrough medications discussed in chapter 8 also turn off these destructive enzymes. When these are successful, permanent joint damage may be delayed or avoided. The sooner these treatments are started before permanent joint damage, the better the results. Fortunately, when identified and treated early, severe crippling deformities occur in less than 5 percent of cases because of new and more effective treatments.

Rheumatoid Arthritis

Rheumatoid arthritis is a serious type of arthritis caused by the body's immune response. Joint pain, swelling, and stiffness can be severe. With rheumatoid arthritis, some of your body's cells recognize a protein as a foreign intruder. The exact protein involved in rheumatoid arthritis has not yet been discovered, and it may be one of a number of possible proteins caused by viral infection, passed on genetically, or present for other reasons. Reacting to this protein are cells called lymphocytes. The reaction causes the release of chemicals called *cytokines,* messengers that trigger more inflammation and destruction from other cells. This battle between the body's chemicals occurs mainly in the joints but can spill over to other areas of the body.

There are many cytokines, but the most important in causing inflammation are tumor necrosis factor (TNF) and interleukin-1. These are thought to trigger many of the other enzymes in rheumatoid arthritis, and because they seem to be the most critical ones, treatments, discussed in chapter 8, are being developed to block these cytokines. Research indicates that blocking these cytokines will also block many of the reactions that damage joints and will help many other arthritis symptoms, such as fatigue.

Because rheumatoid arthritis can cause permanent joint damage, it is sometimes called a crippling disease. In about 20 percent of those with rheumatoid arthritis, lumps—called *rheumatoid nodules*—may develop over joint areas that receive pressure, such as knuckles, elbows, or heels.

Who's at Risk?

Rheumatoid arthritis is the most common type of inflammatory arthritis, with more than 10 million Americans af-

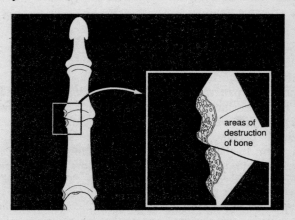

Figure 4.1 An example of bone destruction on a
finger joint caused by rheumatoid arthritis.

fected. More than 70 percent of all rheumatoid arthritis affects women. This serious form of arthritis is most common between ages twenty and fifty, yet even very young children and elderly people can get rheumatoid arthritis.

What You May Feel

Rheumatoid arthritis acts differently than osteoarthritis. The symptoms usually develop gradually but can also start suddenly, and they are more severe than in osteoarthritis. Laura, twenty-eight, woke up feeling feverish, with both knees swollen and stiff—the first sign that something was amiss in her body. Up until that morning, she had felt no pain at all. You may feel pain and stiffness and experience swelling in the following places:

- hands
- wrists
- elbows
- shoulders
- knees
- ankles
- feet
- jaws
- neck

Sometimes this pain occurs in one body part, but it usually occurs in combinations such as in the hands, knees, and feet. In rheumatoid arthritis, the joints tend to be involved in a symmetrical pattern. That is, if the knuckles on the left hand are inflamed, the knuckles on the right hand will also be inflamed. After a period of time, more of your joints may gradually become involved with pain and swelling and may feel warm to the touch. The joint swelling is constant and interferes with the very activities that allow us to function in our daily lives, such as opening a jar, driving, working, and walking.

The stiffness on arising in the morning, which may have been a temporary nuisance, can soon last for hours or even most of the day. You will feel debilitating fatigue, which bothers some people even more than the joint pain. You may lose weight, although your eating habits have not changed. Fever, rash, and even involvement of the heart or lungs can occur.

The symptoms of rheumatoid arthritis may come and go, which we call flares and remissions. Or, your symptoms might just progressively worsen unless controlled with treatments.

Making the Diagnosis

Your doctor will make the diagnosis of rheumatoid arthritis after doing a thorough physical examination, along with x-rays and certain blood tests such as the rheumatoid factor, an indicator of inflammation (page 53) and positive in 70 to 80 percent of those with rheumatoid arthritis. Keep in mind that the rheumatoid factor is not specific for rheumatoid arthritis—meaning you can have a positive result without having rheumatoid arthritis—but it does give your doctor useful information when combined with other signs and symptoms such as pain, swelling, and stiffness.

Although there are many diagnostic tools, x-rays are most helpful in rheumatoid arthritis and can help your doctor detect rheumatoid arthritis in its early stages, when it is very treatable. X-rays of the hands, wrists, and feet are the most useful, because the disease attacks these areas first. X-rays show the first permanent changes in joints and can alert your doctor to start the latest and most effective treatments early in the disease—when treatment is most beneficial and damage is least. The right treatments can actually delay or stop the progress of the bone damage and destruction and can help prevent deformity in the long run. Possible treatment includes the newer breakthrough medications, discussed in chapter 8, along with Super Aspirin, exercises, and moist heat. Treatment must be started early to help prevent much pain, suffering, and expense.

Gout

Daniel, a forty-three-year-old tax attorney, could almost predict the times when he'd suffer with gout. "It never fails but every time I entertain my colleagues or go overboard on food and alcohol, I will have painful gout the next week. I can almost plan my rheumatologist's appointment around my social calendar."

Lucky for Daniel that the new Super Aspirins can give good relief for gout or he'd be staying away from company parties! Once called the "disease of kings," it occurred frequently in the wealthy and royal families. With gout, crystals of uric acid, a normal product of the body's use of protein, rise above normal levels and deposit in the joints, causing inflammation and pain. The crystals may take other forms such as nodules under the skin or stones in the kidney.

Who's at Risk?

Gout can attack after one drinks excessive alcohol. But this common cause of inflammatory arthritis in men over age forty can also develop after surgery or illness or even occur after taking certain medications such as diuretics. Sometimes strict dieting can bring on a gout attack. The painful attacks last several days to a few weeks but can be treated quickly with medications. More than 50 percent of those who have had an acute gouty attack will have a recurrence within the year.

What You May Feel

Gouty arthritis usually strikes suddenly, with severe pain, swelling, warmth, and redness in the large (first) toe in about 75 percent of cases. It causes incapacitating pain that is so severe the weight of bedsheets can cause agonizing distress. Usually one joint is attacked at a time, but there may also be more than one joint affected, including the ankle, knee, wrist, or elbow. The skin over the joint may take on a red or purple shiny appearance. Some people may get kidney stones.

Making the Diagnosis

A high uric acid level in the blood causes gout, which is diagnosed by examining a sample of joint fluid for uric acid crystals. Blood tests can show a high level of uric acid, which increases the chance of gout. Your doctor may prescribe one of the new Super Aspirins along with a medication called Zyloprim (allopurinol) to help end gout attacks.

Systemic Lupus Erythematosus
(SLE, or Lupus)

Systemic lupus erythematosus (SLE or lupus) is another in-flammatory type of arthritis. Like rheumatoid arthritis, the cause of SLE is not known. In SLE, the body reacts to certain proteins that it recognizes as foreign. This reaction, similar to rheumatoid arthritis, causes certain cells to create inflamma-tion by releasing cytokines, which send "messages" to cause arthritis in the joints. Yet with SLE, the inflammation occurs not only in joints but commonly in many internal organs, especially the kidneys, and in the blood vessels, which can cause serious damage to many organs. SLE can also cause fever, rash, heart disease, seizures, blood disorders, and many other life-threatening complications.

Who's at Risk?

More than 90 percent of systemic lupus erythematosus cases in the United States are women. It is most common in younger women, ages twenty to forty, and is more common in African American women.

What You May Feel

With SLE, you will feel pain in many joints, fatigue, and stiffness in the morning. Rashes are common, including the "butterfly rash" across the cheeks in about 15 to 20 percent of cases. An unusual sensitivity to sunlight may develop, causing a rash and other illness. Hair loss, discoloration of the fingers or toes when exposed to cold (Raynaud's phenomenon), and internal organ damage can occur. Half of those with SLE also have kidney disease. Coexisting blood disorders can cause anemia and blood clots. Chest pain from heart and lung inflammation can happen and seizures or strokes can occur.

Making the Diagnosis

Blood tests, especially the antinuclear antibody (ANA) test, can help in diagnosing SLE. About 95 percent of active cases of SLE have a positive ANA blood test, although everyone with a positive test does not have SLE. ANAs are found in patients whose immune system is prone to cause inflammation against their own body tissues. Once your doctor evaluates the clinical findings and blood tests from the examination, she can decide if your symptoms suggest SLE and start you on the proper treatment.

Polymyalgia Rheumatica

Polymyalgia rheumatica is a type of arthritis with inflammation felt mainly around the joints rather than only in the joints themselves. There may be mild swelling in the hands or shoulders, but pain and stiffness are the main problems.

Who's at Risk?

This disease usually affects people over age fifty (or, more commonly, older than sixty). There is no known cause, and it often occurs in those who are otherwise in good health.

What You May Feel

With polymyalgia rheumatica, you may feel a sudden or gradual onset of severe pain and stiffness in the muscles around the shoulders, upper arms, hips, and thighs. There is usually no joint swelling, but you may have severe fatigue and stiffness when you get out of bed in the morning. You may also run a fever, lose weight, or have a poor appetite.

Making the Diagnosis

Your doctor will test your blood sedimentation rate, which will be very high in polymyalgia rheumatica. You will also be tested for other diseases that can mimic polymyalgia rheumatica. Temporal arteritis, a disease caused by inflammation in the arteries, may travel along with polymyalgia rheumatica. A proper diagnosis is important to begin treatment early and prevent complications such as loss of vision. Super Aspirins may be used for polymyalgia rheumatica, along with low doses of prednisone.

Ankylosing Spondylitis

Will has lived with ankylosing spondylitis as long as he can remember, and two of his sons, ages twelve and fourteen, were just diagnosed with it as well. This type of arthritis attacks the joints of the spine and usually starts gradually as lower back pain. The hallmark feature of ankylosing spondylitis (AS) is the involvement of the joints at the base of the spine where the spine joins the pelvis—the sacroiliac joints.

Who's at Risk?

Ankylosing spondylitis strikes more than 300,000 people, the majority of whom are men. It is most common in young men, especially from the teen years to age thirty. About 95 percent of those with AS have a positive blood test for HLA-B27 antigen. If a parent has AS and carries the B27 genetic factor, the children have about a one-in-five chance of developing the disease themselves. Even girls who may have inherited this gene (and 50 percent will have it), may develop AS.

What You May Feel

Ankylosing spondylitis usually starts gradually as pain in the lower back that may come and go at first. Instead of improving, as would be expected from an injury or strain, it gradually worsens. The lower back pain may gradually work its way up the spine. You may even mistake your AS for an injury, but the pain does not go away.

The most common site of pain is in the lower back and buttocks. You may also feel pain farther up the back, perhaps between the shoulder blades and in the neck. You will also feel stiffness and pain in your back on arising in the morning, more pain when resting, and less pain if some activity is continued. After five to ten years, you may have pain in the middle back, then the upper back, then your neck. The pain and stiffness continue, but as the disease progresses, your spine may stiffen and become difficult to bend for usual daily activities such as walking, lifting, and driving.

Making the Diagnosis

X-rays of the back can help clinch the diagnosis of ankylosing spondylitis, along with a positive blood test for HLA-B27 antigen. This test suggests that the patient has a higher than usual chance of developing arthritis in the spine. The sooner the diagnosis, the earlier treatment can begin to help prevent any spine deformity.

Arthritis Caused by Infections

Infections can also cause arthritis. A joint infection is most likely to occur following a previous infection elsewhere in the body. The germ travels to the joint via the bloodstream after it has entered the body through a person's skin, nose, throat, or ears. These are the most common entry points, but sometimes the germ may enter through an existing wound. There is usually only one joint involved and it is mainly the large ones—shoulders, hips, or knees—that are affected. However, sometimes two or three joints can become infected and smaller joints can be involved, although less frequently.

Infectious arthritis is usually not a long-term illness. In most cases, it can be cured if treated promptly and properly. Without treatment, there is a risk of serious damage to the affected joints, and the infection can spread to other parts of the body.

Who's at Risk?

People who are at greatest risk for infectious arthritis include those who have:

- diabetes
- sickle-cell anemia
- kidney disease
- staph infection
- gonorrhea
- AIDS and HIV
- immune deficiency
- some forms of cancer
- alcoholism
- intravenous drug abuse

Staphylococcus bacteria can cause a very serious form of arthritis. If this staph attacks a joint, it can cause severe damage within days if left untreated. Usually staph infections attack only one joint (usually the knee, wrist, or ankle) and may frequently appear after injury or skin infection.

Lyme Disease

Lyme disease (Lyme arthritis) is a recently discovered type of infectious arthritis caused by the *Borrelia burgdorferi* organism. It is most common in the spring and summer months, when field mice and deer carry this organism and pass it on to ticks. The ticks bite humans, resulting in a host of flulike symptoms. You may not even realize you were bitten by a tick when the symptoms hit.

There are specific stages of Lyme disease, and each stage has its own signs and symptoms.

Stage 1: This occurs days to months after the tick bite. You may have a rash (called *erythema chronicum migrans*) on the groin or other area. This rash will become larger, and you may have other rashes on your body. You may have flulike feelings such as headache, joint and muscle pain, fever, chills, sore throat, stiff neck, and fatigue. Blood tests may be negative and leave your doctor puzzled about what ails you.

Stage 2: About 10 percent of those with Lyme disease move on to stage 2. At this point, the nerves are involved, and you'll have headaches and feel weak. Bell's palsy (facial weakness) can occur at this point, and heart disease occurs in approximately 10 percent of those infected. Blood tests for detection may still be negative at stage 2.

Stage 3: After a period of several years, some people with Lyme disease hit stage 3, characterized by chronic arthritis pain, stiffness, and swelling in the joints. This stage mimics rheumatoid arthritis, yet now the doctor can make a positive diagnosis using blood tests.

For all stages of Lyme disease, antibiotics are the standard form of treatment. Especially if given in the early stages, antibiotics such as penicillin or tetracycline work well. However, if you have heart problems or arthritis symptoms, high doses of penicillin or other antibiotics are necessary.

Other Inflammatory Types

Psoriatic Arthritis

Psoriatic arthritis is a less common type of inflammatory arthritis. But like rheumatoid arthritis, it can cause deformity and crippling, so it is important to treat it early and effectively.

Psoriatic arthritis affects both men and women, usually between the ages of twenty and fifty, and occurs in 10 percent or more of people who have the skin disease psoriasis.

The reason that some people with psoriasis develop arthritis is not known. Psoriasis causes rashes, which can be thick, scaly skin over the knees, elbows, or other areas. The other symptoms of psoriatic arthritis are similar to rheumatoid arthritis, and more than 80 percent of people will also have pitted or thickened nails. You'll also have morning stiffness and fatigue, just as with rheumatoid arthritis. You may have pain and stiffness in the hands, wrists, elbows, shoulders, knees, ankles, feet, and spine.

Your doctor can make this diagnosis based on a physical examination, patient history, and laboratory tests. The treatment for psoriatic arthritis is similar to that for rheumatoid arthritis, including the use of moist heat, exercises, NSAIDs, and Super Aspirins or other medications discussed in chapters 7 and 8.

Scleroderma

Scleroderma, or "hard skin," is a serious form of arthritis that has no known cause. With this type, there is an overproduction of collagen, which is a building block of skin and other structures in your body. The collagen replaces normal tissues so those affected quit living functionally the way they should. The blood supply to these organs is also decreased.

Scleroderma is more common in women than men, but the reasons are not known. With scleroderma, you may experience discoloration and pain in your fingers when they are cold, known as Raynaud's phenomenon. As the disease progresses, the skin can thicken and harden so that your body structures actually appear frozen in one position. Your fingers may lose their blood supply. Ulcers may form on your skin, and it will easily tear and break. Scleroderma becomes life-threatening when the lungs or kidneys are involved.

After a proper diagnosis, your doctor will work to treat and minimize the symptoms and control pain. There is no cure for scleroderma right now, but your doctor can help you with newer treatments of antibiotics that may help control the disease.

Sjögren's Syndrome

This type of arthritis commonly occurs with other types of arthritis, usually rheumatoid arthritis. Although the cause is unknown, it is common in women, and more than 50 percent of those with Sjögren's also have rheumatoid or another type of arthritis.

Because the glands in the eyes and mouth do not give adequate moisture (tears or saliva), you will experience dryness of the eyes and mouth. The parotid glands on the sides of the face may swell, and internal organ diseases and blood abnormalities may occur.

Your doctor may make the diagnosis after talking with you and after a physical examination. A simple biopsy of the lip or other area and examination by an ophthalmologist can confirm the diagnosis.

Vasculitis

In vasculitis, the blood vessels (particularly the arteries) are damaged by abnormal proteins circulating in the blood. When this happens, some organs lose their oxygen and nutrient supply, causing damage. Although the causes of vasculitis are not well understood, many believe the body's immune system starts to damage blood vessels in the same manner it attacks other foreign invaders in the body.

This type of arthritis can attack at any age. It can also complicate other diseases and infections, such as hepatitis and serious bloodstream infections. Vasculitis can occur in conjunction with other diseases such as rheumatoid arthritis or SLE.

Although symptoms may begin as a rash and joint pain or stiffness, they can progress to more serious and irreversible organ damage. Sometimes the fingers turn white on exposure to cold, as in scleroderma. You may even have gangrene in the fingers and toes from poor circulation. The kidneys, lungs, and heart may also be involved.

Proper diagnosis is imperative if vasculitis is suspected.

Your doctor will do a biopsy of an organ or x-ray of the arteries to help with a correct diagnosis. The outlook for this disease is good, if early treatment using cortisone drugs or other medications are used.

Childhood Arthritis

Chronic childhood arthritis is often called juvenile rheumatoid arthritis, although it is quite different from adult rheumatoid arthritis. Many have dropped the word *rheumatoid* and now call chronic childhood arthritis juvenile arthritis, or JA.

Approximately one in one thousand children under the age of sixteen suffers from arthritis, making the ailment more common than most chronic childhood disorders, including diabetes or cystic fibrosis. JA is more common in girls, who account for 85 percent of juvenile rheumatoid arthritis cases.

What Your Child May Feel

With JA the immune system is overactive, causing continuous inflammation. This inflammation results in warm, stiff, swollen, and often painful joints. If your child has JA, he may avoid certain activities or complain about pains in his joints.

If your child has these symptoms, have the doctor check it out. Although these symptoms may be "growing pains," sometimes they indicate arthritis, which can cause swelling, pain, immobility, and inflammation, even in the eyes. Your doctor will look carefully for any signs of joint swelling or loss of mobility that suggest that the joints are inflamed. Also with JA, your child's growth will be monitored to make sure it is even and normal. Sometimes a child with JA may suffer from chronic uveitis, which is an inflammation inside the eye that may hinder vision. As with all types of arthritis, it is important to have your doctor evaluate your child frequently until this type of arthritis is controlled with treatment.

....

CHAPTER 5

Making the Diagnosis: Tests You May Need

"Doc, my back is killing me!" many patients say when they come to my clinics. Next to the common cold, back pain is the most common reason people visit their doctors. In fact, 80 percent of us have had back pain at some time in our lives; 50 percent of all adults suffer with back pain each year.

If you have arthritis, back pain is a frequent complaint. You may also complain of painful and stiff joints in the knees, ankles, hips, neck, shoulders, hands, or feet. Arthritis pain can throb or it can be vague and difficult to pinpoint, such as with the deep muscle pain or the trigger, or tender, points of fibromyalgia. Some types of arthritis pain can produce sensations of numbness or weakness in the legs, feet, hands, and fingers. In the more serious inflammatory types of arthritis, you may even have symptoms of internal organ disease involving the heart or lungs.

No matter where you hurt, many different problems can create these painful feelings, and a proper diagnosis is essential to treat it effectively. Take Mike, for example. This forty-seven-year-old attorney and weekend warrior was playing in an amateur tennis tournament several months ago. As he twisted his body to use his new backhand swing, he felt excruciating lower-back pain he described as a "blowtorch down the spine.'' Initially the pain was sharp and penetrating, pulsating down his right leg like an electrical shock—enough to make Mike forfeit his game. Interestingly, this pain worsened when he sat in a chair and decreased when he stood up. Within hours of the injury, his right leg and foot felt numb; that night he was unable to sleep due to severe pain.

Mike assumed this pain was the result of arthritis. After all, he was over forty, and his father had osteoarthritis in his hips and knees. So Mike decided to treat himself, as many people do. He rested in bed a few days, using regular compresses of ice on his back to reduce the inflammation and alleviate the pain. He then tried to continue his usual routine at work. After three weeks, Mike felt no improvement. In fact, he said that because he was sleeping so poorly, he was ineffective with his clients. That's when he called me for an evaluation.

After we discussed his symptoms, I gave Mike a physical examination and used a special test called magnetic resonance imaging (MRI), described on page 56. I found that Mike *did* have osteoarthritis in his lower back. But I also discovered that Mike's back pain was *not* caused by arthritis; instead it resulted from a ruptured disc in his lower lumbar spine. Because he had no improvement and the pain was interfering with his activity, Mike planned surgery to remove the ruptured disc material and since the operation he has had no pain.

For those who experience unending pain like Mike's or notice any new pain and swelling, a diagnosis is necessary to discern the actual cause of the problem so that proper treatment can end the pain.

Seeking a Diagnosis

The diagnosis of arthritis is made after discussion and a physical examination with your internist, arthritis specialist (rheumatologist), or primary care physician. He or she will start by obtaining a detailed medical history, including any information on symptoms, how you feel, your activity level and diet, your home and work environment, and family history, and then do a thorough medical examination.

During this examination, it is important that you openly discuss how you've been feeling and what symptoms you've been experiencing so your doctor can factor this into the results of the physical examination, the laboratory testing, and x-rays. I've had many patients who waited until every test was exhausted to tell me that their pain kept them from sleeping or working. Be upfront with your doctor, and describe your symptoms accurately and thoroughly. Some of my patients write them down and bring their list to the appointment, saying it helps them remember everything. In the long run, honest communication will save you time and money, because your diagnosis will be easier to make.

In this chapter, I describe the tests commonly used to diagnose the various types of arthritis. Trust your doctor to decide which set of tests is best in your case to ensure no other medical problems are present. If you still do not feel comfortable with the diagnosis, talk to your doctor and have more testing done. Or, get a second opinion, to help you to feel sure that the problem has been diagnosed correctly. Remember, this is *your* body and *your* pain!

Gaining control of your arthritis depends on an accurate diagnosis. Keep in mind that there is usually no "official" order of tests. Your doctor may order an x-ray first, while another specialist may do a complete blood count initially. Once the type of arthritis is properly identified, your doctor can prescribe a treatment regimen that helps to reduce pain and stiffness and increase mobility.

Blood Tests

For most types of arthritis, such as rheumatoid arthritis or SLE (systemic lupus erythematosus), a few blood tests can either confirm the type of arthritis or rule out many other types. However, for osteoarthritis—the most common arthritis—and fibromyalgia, bursitis, and tendinitis, there are no specific blood test abnormalities, but usually some tests are necessary to be sure no other problems or conditions are present. If medication is being considered, blood tests will ensure that there are no preexisting problems and that your kidneys and liver test in a normal, healthy range. Thyroid tests are often performed on arthritis patients, because an overactive or underactive thyroid can aggravate the signs and symptoms of many types of arthritis.

Complete Blood Count (CBC) and Blood Chemistry Tests

Your doctor may take a sample of your blood for a complete blood count (CBC) and chemical profile. These results will help assess your general health and identify any other diseases that you may have along with arthritis. The CBC measures the amount of red and white blood cells and shows how your vital organs such as your kidneys and liver are functioning. Your doctor can tell from the white cells and platelet count whether you are anemic or have an infection. A high level of uric acid in the blood may indicate the presence of gout.

Sedimentation Rate and Rheumatoid Factor

Your doctor may also do a blood test that shows the sedimentation rate (also called sed rate), which measures inflammation in the body. The sedimentation rate can be high in almost any type of inflammatory arthritis, but in osteoarthritis, the rheumatoid factor is negative, and the sed rate is usually near normal. If the sed rate is elevated, it is an indication that you may have an inflammatory-type arthritis. Seventy-five to eighty percent of patients with rheumatoid arthritis have elevated sed rates. But a high sed rate is not present in all cases and can actually be present in other types of arthritis or even in otherwise normal people. This is an important test to help diagnose the type of arthritis.

Antinuclear Antibody (ANA)

The antinuclear antibody (ANA) is an abnormal protein found in blood testing. It's an important test for lupus, because it's found in 95 percent of active cases of SLE. But a few cases will be negative, and ANA can be positive for other kinds of arthritis and even in otherwise healthy people. Some medications or viral infections can cause a patient without SLE to test positive. But if the ANA is positive, other more specific tests can be ordered to help determine whether other varieties of SLE-like illnesses are present. Your internist or arthritis specialist can guide you.

Joint Fluid Test

Different types of arthritis may cause different changes in the joint fluid. Most arthritis causes swelling in the joints, which is a result of excess fluid production or swelling of the joint lining. Removing a sample of the joint fluid with a small needle under local anesthesia can be a quick, safe, almost painless, and inexpensive way to quickly find out what's causing your arthritis.

Normal joints contain a very small amount of joint fluid, and it is usually a yellow, almost clear, and somewhat thick (viscous) fluid that drips slowly from a needle.

With osteoarthritis, the joint fluid usually looks normal (not cloudy), but it's increased in amount. With rheumatoid arthritis, the fluid is usually more cloudy and much thinner, and there may be more fluid than normal. With gout, the fluid is often cloudy and has crystals in it, which can be seen under a special polarized microscope. In arthritis caused by infection in the joints, a sample of the joint fluid can quickly diagnose the infection that could damage or destroy the joint if left untreated.

Imaging Tests

The following imaging tests are commonly used to assess the type of arthritis.

X-rays

Your doctor may begin with x-rays of the affected joints. In osteoarthritis, x-rays will let your doctor see the changes in the joints with narrowing of the cartilage space as shown on page 21. On an x-ray, there are often spurs—extra bone growths called *osteophytes*—which usually can be seen by the time you seek medical treatment.

In bursitis and tendinitis some minor changes may be apparent on an x-ray, including calcium deposits around the painful joint, but it's more likely that the x-rays will be completely normal. If another type of arthritis is present, such as rheumatoid arthritis, it might also show up on an x-ray even though the initial problem is bursitis or tendinitis. In fibromyalgia, no changes in the joints are visible on an x-ray, though doctors may order x-rays to be sure no other problems are present. Unless there is a secondary type of arthritis, x-rays are normal in fibromyalgia.

In rheumatoid arthritis, x-rays are important to make an accurate diagnosis and will predict how the arthritis might improve or worsen in the future. Although in early cases of rheumatoid arthritis, the diagnosis is difficult to make, treatment is most effective if the diagnosis is made early in the disease (see chapter 8) and prevents permanent damage to the joints. X-rays can show the earliest changes in the joints, which appear as tiny erosions at the edges of the bones of the hands, wrists, and feet (page 37). The erosions on x-rays are a red flag indicating that a more serious form of rheumatoid arthritis might be brewing, one that could become crippling as it progresses, and they signal the need for early and aggressive treatment with effective medications to prevent long-term damage and deformity. Available medications can slow down or stop the progress of the arthritis in the bones before there are any outward or visible signs of severe arthritis.

X-rays can also diagnose arthritis in the spine in cases of back pain. X-rays of the lower (lumbar) spine are an easy way to examine the bones in this area. The most common type of arthritis in the spine is osteoarthritis, with the x-ray showing narrowing of the cartilage discs between the vertebral bones and spurs along the spine. Yet other types of arthritis can attack the spine. For example, ankylosing spondylitis causes calcium bridges to form between the bones of the spine. The spine becomes stiffened starting at the lower back and gradually working up to the neck over five to ten years. This can usually be found on x-ray of the lower back and is an important sign that allows for early treatment to prevent deformity.

It is important to refrain from using x-rays prematurely to limit your exposure to radiation. And remember that although x-rays can detect arthritis, cancer, fractures in the spine, and some infections, they *cannot* detect a ruptured disc.

Magnetic Resonance Imaging (MRI)

Magnetic resonance imaging (MRI) can be used to evaluate the knee, the shoulder, the spine, or other areas, because this test reveals abnormalities of cartilage and ligaments that routine x-rays cannot. But MRIs aren't used routinely because of their cost. If your doctor suspects that your shoulder or knee pain is caused by a torn ligament or damaged cartilage, MRI may be used to confirm it.

MRI can reveal the cause of severe back pain, showing osteoarthritis, other types of arthritis in the spine, and ruptured discs, common in osteoarthritis patients, with more than 95 percent accuracy. Ruptured discs can cause back pain to travel down a leg and can be severely limiting. MRI can also show lumbar stenosis, narrowing of the spinal canal that contains nerve roots coming from the spinal cord (see page

32). Once the diagnosis is made, effective treatment with medications or surgery can begin.

Because it does not involve radiation, MRI is safe and can be done as an outpatient procedure. With the older types of MRI, you are placed in a long, nonmagnetic tube, which is surrounded by a huge doughnut-shaped magnet. The entire procedure lasts from thirty to ninety minutes. Newer, open types of MRI are preferred by many patients to avoid the closed-in feeling of the narrow tubelike opening of the older-style machines. This test is not done on patients who have had metal implants such as artificial joints or pacemakers, because the metal interferes with the images.

Computed Tomographic Scan (CT Scan)

A computed tomographic scan (CT scan) is also used for severe back pain caused by arthritis. It can detect a ruptured disc in more than 90 percent of cases in the lumbar spine but can occasionally suggest an abnormality when the disc is actually normal. A CT scan is more accurate than an x-ray to find infection, fracture of a bone, or cancer. With an acceptable level of radiation exposure, CT is done as an outpatient procedure and is less confining than MRI for those who have a fear of being closed in.

Bone Scan

A bone scan is used mainly when your doctor may suspect something more than arthritis is going on, such as infection, cancer, or a bone fracture. The scan can detect abnormal areas of bone produced by these problems in any part of the skeleton. The test is painless except for the injection of a small amount of radioactive dye into a vein in the arm followed in a few hours by a scan of the body while the patient lies on an x-ray table.

Myelogram

For those with severe back pain that mimics both osteoarthritis and a ruptured disc, a doctor may use a myelogram to confirm the diagnosis. This special x-ray requires an injection of dye into the spinal canal through a lumbar needle to show the rupture of a disc or other problems. Normally the dye would fill the spinal canal, as well as the nerve root sheaths, giving a revealing outline for an x-ray. Yet an abnormal myelogram shows an absence of dye in a specific area. This is called a filling defect and indicates that the nerve root or spinal cord is pinched or compressed. This test detects the rupture in more than 95 percent of cases.

Compared to MRI, the myelogram has more discomfort, requires an injection, and has a greater possibility of an unwanted side effect such as a headache. Some experts now first recommend MRI of the lumbar spine; if this fails to provide a clear answer, a myelogram is performed. A CT scan may be combined with a myelogram to improve the accuracy of the diagnosis, especially if a small piece of disc has broken off and is pressing on a nerve away from its root between the vertebrae.

Discogram

Your doctor may recommend a discogram to see if a ruptured disc is actually the cause of your back pain. You lie facedown on the procedure table, and, using three-dimensional imaging under radio-television control, the surgeon will inject dye into the disc rupture. Radiographic films are taken; then, after a short period, the needles are removed. If the film shows that dye leaks out of the disc, your doctor will know that the disc is ruptured. This test is often combined with a CT scan for greater accuracy.

Electromyelogram (EMG)

Severe back pain and arthritis may make it difficult to diagnose the exact cause, but an electromyelogram (EMG) may help your doctor accurately diagnose your pain. The EMG measures the electrical activity in the muscles supplied by the nerves that are being irritated by a ruptured or herniated disc. A nerve conduction study tests the velocity at which the nerve transmits its signal. In other words, if the nerve is pinched, its ability to transmit a signal is reduced. Abnormal muscle activity and slowed nerve conduction both suggest a pinched or irritated nerve from a disc rupture.

Arthrogram

In this test, dye is injected into a joint to show the structures in greater detail. An arthrogram can be painful, so it is not used very often because MRI may give similar information without as much discomfort.

Why Diagnostic Tests Are Important

I see many patients who hesitate to have further testing when arthritis is suspected. "Can't I just take a Super Aspirin and see if it works?" they ask. My response is that different types of arthritis warrant different types of treatment. Your doctor may assume you have rheumatoid arthritis after examining the painful swelling in your knees, ankles, and feet, because these are typical symptoms. Yet these are also symptoms of gout, another form of arthritis that has a different cause and treatment. Unless the joint fluid is examined under a polarized microscope, a correct diagnosis may not be made. This confusion could result in delayed treatment, because gout and rheumatoid arthritis are two different diseases. Gout is easily treated—and prevented—and can be controlled in almost all cases once the diagnosis is made. It often takes time and more powerful medications to regain control of the symptoms of rheumatoid arthritis.

Let me share Terri's story. When she was in her mid-forties, Terri's family doctor had diagnosed her with osteoarthritis and had prescribed a traditional NSAID for pain and swelling in her knees and hands, especially at the base of her thumbs. Yet a few months after this diagnosis, her arthritis worsened, with more swelling in her hands and wrists. When Terri came to see me, I listened to her describe the new pain and knew that it was similar to that of rheumatoid arthritis—severe stiffness in the morning, difficulty walking and doing daily tasks, and not being able to work because of tremendous swelling in her feet and ankles. Although her family doctor's diagnosis of osteoarthritis was accurate, Terri had also developed rheumatoid arthritis, which I diagnosed after seeing the subtle, telltale changes on the x-rays of her hands. Terri did not improve until she was treated with methotrexate, a medicine for rheumatoid arthritis (discussed in chapter 8), which does not help osteoarthritis.

Controlling your arthritis starts with an accurate diagnosis. Once the type of arthritis is properly identified, your doctor can prescribe a treatment regimen that includes Super Aspirins or another breakthrough medication along with exercises, moist heat, and other healing approaches that will work together to end your arthritis pain.

CHAPTER 6

What's Wrong with Aspirin and NSAIDs?

The experience of arthritis pain—from the dull ache of an arthritic hip, to the misery of back pain, to the swollen and stiff hands of rheumatoid arthritis—is universal. If you suffer with arthritis pain, you've probably lived on aspirin or NSAIDs to end pain and stiffness and to allow you to be active. The effects of traditional arthritis medications are beneficial, yet frequently the side effects, especially gastrointestinal problems, create more trouble than you bargained for.

In 1997, Americans consumed more than $2.5 billion worth of over-the-counter analgesics (pain relievers). Although these medications relieve pain, swelling, and stiffness, can they be taken without side effects? Probably not. Aspirin and traditional NSAIDs may injure your stomach lining, cause gastrointestinal bleeding or ulcers, and even cause kidney damage. For older patients and those who need full doses of or as many as ten NSAIDs daily to control pain, stomach problems frequently cause more complications than the arthritis itself. And some analgesics like acetaminophen can cause liver damage if taken in excess or with alcohol.

So what's wrong with regular aspirin and NSAIDs are the side effects. Here are some facts and statistics.

- If you use NSAIDs, you have a 30 percent chance of incurring stomach or intestinal damage.

- About one-half of those who sustain stomach damage will develop peptic ulcers.

- Peptic ulcers may be silent and produce no symptoms.

- Of the 13 million Americans who take NSAIDs to treat arthritis and pain, up to 100,000 are hospitalized each year from complications caused by the drugs, such as ulcers, bleeding, and small perforations most without warning signs.

- More than 17,000 people die every year from aspirin- or NSAID-induced gastrointestinal side effects.

The NSAID/Ulcer Connection

The documented NSAID/ulcer connection is all too common. One of my patients, Lorri, a forty-nine-year-old mother of three, was rushed to the crowded emergency room with excruciating stomach pain in the middle of the night. For weeks, she had been living on aspirin for osteoarthritis pain in her knees, yet had noticed an increase in stomach upset with heartburn, belching, and bloating. By the time Lorri got to the hospital, she was in tremendous pain, and the staff wondered if she needed emergency surgery. After a series of tests, it was determined that she had a gastric ulcer. The good news is that once Lorri got off the aspirin and began taking Tagamet, a medication that blocks acid in the stomach, she recovered. The bad news? Without the NSAID, Lorri's arthritis pain skyrocketed, and she was unable to be as active as she liked.

A fifty-one-year-old patient named Ralph developed severe heartburn after taking ibuprofen for arthritis. This NSAID had helped relieve Ralph's constant pain from osteoarthritis of the hip, enabling him to walk several miles a day—without pain or stiffness. At first he managed his heartburn with antacids—medications that counteract stomach acid. Nonetheless, one day his pain was so severe that he felt short of breath and was having severe chest pains. Ralph took Tums, but the pain worsened, and taking a few more did not help at all. When he finally got to our clinic, he was in so much pain that I wondered if he was having a heart attack, because the symptoms are often similar.

I diagnosed Ralph with a duodenal ulcer and gave him Tagamet to help it heal. Though his arthritic hips hurt more because he had to stop taking ibuprofen, he did feel relieved to have no more heartburn or stomach pain.

Because NSAIDs reduce the stomach's natural protection from acid damage, most people will pop Tums or another antacid to relieve the heartburn. Although antacids are excellent medications for occasional heartburn, they do not prevent peptic ulcers when you take NSAIDs. In fact, most people who have intestinal bleeding or perforation of the stomach have no early warning symptoms. Especially in older people, the first sign could be when bleeding starts, which leads to hospitalization and an increased risk of complications.

Traditional Pain Relievers

To see why Super Aspirins are a miraculous breakthrough in treating pain, let's look at the pain medications traditionally used for arthritis.

Aspirin

"Take two aspirins, and call me in the morning." For years, this has been a common recommendation for anyone who complained of aches and pains. Since its discovery more than one hundred years ago, traditional aspirin has been the main treatment for arthritis sufferers. In fact, Americans, choosing from more than fifty over-the-counter products, consume more than 30 billion aspirin tablets annually. All together, aspirin and other NSAIDs such as ibuprofen, naproxen, and ketoprofen are used daily by approximately 30 million people worldwide, constituting a world market in excess of $2.5 billion.

As early as the fifth century B.C., Hippocrates prescribed a bitter powder from the bark of a willow tree to treat aches and pains. In the eighteenth century, Edmund Stone, an Anglican clergyman, discovered the healing effects of willow bark—a substance called salicyclic acid. Aspirin as we know it today was developed in 1897 by chemist Felix Hoffmann, who compounded the pill of acetylsalicyclic acid to treat his father's rheumatism pain.

Since aspirin became the standard arthritis treatment, many people have taken twelve to fourteen aspirins every day to control pain and swelling. Although a lower dose can help relieve pain, it won't stop inflammation. And even low doses of aspirin, even when enteric coated or buffered, can still cause stomach problems and intestinal bleeding. The higher dose often worked well for arthritis, but the most common side effects were upset stomach and ringing in the ears (tinnitus). At these doses, the upset stomach can lead to abdominal pain and nausea, plus a pretty good chance of a peptic ulcer and intestinal bleeding. So for decades, many people faced a tradeoff: control their arthritis, but risk dangerous side effects.

Through the years, research began to show that aspirin has additional beneficial effects. It lowers the risk of heart attack in men by preventing platelets in the blood from sticking together to form a blood clot, which often causes a heart attack. Aspirin also lowers the risk of colon cancer and may lower the risk of Alzheimer's disease and cataracts.

Acetaminophen

Acetaminophen (Tylenol) is a pain reliever—not a traditional NSAID. Many doctors prescribe this drug for pain that does *not* stem from inflammation, because it does not affect prostaglandins. So it's the only pain reliever that does not cause stomach upset and gastrointestinal bleeding, but it does not reduce inflammation in arthritis. This pain reliever is often tried first in osteoarthritis, and although it may work for a few months because it's a good treatment for mild to moderate pain, most people need more than acetaminophen for relief. If taken with alcohol, acetaminophen can cause liver damage.

Nonsteroid Anti-Inflammatory Drugs (NSAIDs)

Other than aspirin, NSAIDs are the most heavily used drugs in the world. These medications work as anti-inflammatory agents and pain relievers. In 1997 more than 77 million prescriptions were written for NSAIDs, and this number doesn't include the millions of over-the-counter NSAIDs taken by the American public.

Developed in the early 1960s, NSAIDs, like aspirin, block prostaglandin production. NSAIDs include such over-the-counter products as Advil and Motrin (ibuprofen), Actron and Orudis KT (ketoprofen), and Aleve (naproxen). NSAIDs are nonaddictive and do not usually cause sedation or respiratory problems. The ibuprofen pain relief usually lasts for four to six hours, while naproxen lasts for seven to eight hours in most people.

Today there are more than fifty NSAIDs available. These drugs give the benefits of high-dose aspirin with fewer side effects. With each one there is variation in individual responses to pain control and the possibility of side effects. Yet although these traditional NSAIDs can relieve pain and stiffness, they still can cause stomach problems and kidney damage.

Before you take any medication, be sure to read the package insert for side effects, as well as any drug-drug or drug-food interactions that could occur. The dosage of each medicine may differ, depending on the type of medicine and strength. Ask your doctor or pharmacist for the correct dosage for your specific problem. Taking an NSAID with a meal may help prevent stomach problems.

COMMONLY USED ANALGESICS

BRAND NAME	GENERIC
Advil	ibuprofen
Aleve	naproxen
Anacin	aspirin
Anacin-3	acetaminophen
Anacin Maximum Strength	aspirin
Ascriptin, buffered aspirin	aspirin
Bayer	aspirin
Bufferin	buffered aspirin
Excedrin Extra Strength	aspirin, acetaminophen
Motrin IB	ibuprofen
Norwich	aspirin
Nuprin	ibuprofen
Orudis	ketoprofen
Panex	acetaminophen
Tylenol	acetaminophen
Vanquish	aspirin, acetaminophen

COMMONLY USED NONSTEROID ANTI-INFLAMMATORY DRUGS (NSAIDs) FOR PAIN AND INFLAMMATION

BRAND NAME	GENERIC
Advil	ibuprofen
Aleve	naproxen
Anaprox	naproxen
Ansaid	flurbiprofen
Arthrotec	diclofenac and misoprostol
Aspirin Products	aspirin
Cataflam	diclofenac
Clinoril	sulindac
Daypro	oxaprozin
Disalcid, Salflex, Mono-Gesic	salsalate
Dolobid	diflunisal
Feldene	piroxicam
Indocin	indomethacin
Lodine	etodolac
Magan	magnesium salicylate
Meclomen	meclofenamate
Nalfon	fenoprofen
Naprosyn EC	naproxen (enteric-coated)
Naprelan	naproxen
Naprosyn	naproxen
Oruvail	ketoprofen (delayed release)
Relafen	nabumetone
Tolectin	tolmetin
Trilisate	choline magnesium trisalicylate
Voltaren	diclofenac
Zorprin	twelve-hour aspirin

The Downside of NSAIDs

Although NSAIDs relieve pain and swelling, they can have serious side effects. Traditional NSAIDs such as aspirin, ibuprofen, and naproxen or any of the others increase the risk of hospitalization and death from gastrointestinal bleeding or stomach or intestinal perforation from peptic ulcer. It is not unusual for arthritis patients to take as many as ten or more aspirin daily to relieve pain and stiffness. Yet in doing so, they risk abdominal pain, nausea, peptic ulcers, and bleeding from the stomach or intestine as possible side effects. Aspirin may cause you to bleed or bruise easily, and as many as one in five asthma patients have breathing problems after taking this product due to allergy. Other symptoms associated with NSAIDs are listed in the box.

Side Effects of NSAIDs

....

Abdominal pain	Indigestion
Abnormal liver tests (blood tests)	Intestinal bleeding
	Lower hemoglobin (anemia)
Asthma in those allergic to NSAIDs	Decrease of platelet effect (can affect bleeding)
Aggravation of or kidney (renal) failure	Interaction with or change of effect of other medication
Diminished effect of diuretics	
Dizziness	Peptic ulcer
Gastritis	Ringing in the ears (tinnitus)
Heartburn	
Increased blood pressure (hypertension)	

Less Common Side Effects

Confusion

Constipation

Depression

Diarrhea

Difficulty in sleeping

Fatigue

Headaches

Impaired thinking
(uncommon, but occurs at
times in older patients)

Itching

Lowered white blood cell
count

Meningitislike illness (rare)

Mouth ulcers

Occasional blurred vision

Other individual allergic or
unusual reactions

Palpitations

Rash

Sodium retention with
edema (swelling)

Sun sensitivity

Often No Warning

It's important to keep in mind that most of those who are admitted to a hospital for an NSAID-related complication have *no prior warning symptoms*. These serious and sometimes fatal side effects are more common in patients sixty-five years or older who take these medicines, but they can happen to anyone. Take Ellen, for example. This middle-aged woman had been taking a prescription NSAID for four years. She had never experienced stomach pain and could not remember ever having had heartburn—until one morning at work.

I was sitting at my desk drinking coffee and trying to finish a report my boss needed immediately. I had taken my medicine early that morning, then had not eaten breakfast, which I usually do. By nine A.M., I had already downed three strong cups of coffee. Then around ten A.M., I felt a stabbing pain in my stomach that almost knocked me over. I quickly drank some cold water, thinking that would resolve it, but it kept coming strong. Finally, I was in such agony, I had a co-worker drive me to the emergency room. I thought I was dying.

Ellen stayed in the hospital for four days while diagnostic tests were done, and we finally diagnosed her with a bleeding peptic ulcer. She had to put away her arthritis medication and start taking Prilosec (omeprazole) to help block stomach acid and allow her painful ulcer to heal.

If you are careful to watch for side effects, sometimes NSAIDs can be taken over a long period of time. If your doctor wants you to stay on an NSAID, see if a medication that reduces acid and may protect the stomach lining and prevent peptic ulcers would be helpful. The following medications are taken differently, depending on the severity of your stomach problem. Available both over the counter and by prescription are Axid, Pepcid AC, Tagamet, and Zantac; available by prescription only are Cytotec, Prevacid, and Prilosec. Your doctor can prescribe the most effective medication and treatment regimen.

CHAPTER 7

The Super Aspirin Cure
for Arthritis: COX-2 Inhibitors

Our group of rheumatologists has known for years from our patients that we need new medicines to stop inflammation without damaging the stomach. Yet all we've had to prescribe are varying derivatives of aspirin or traditional NSAIDs and acetaminophen.

So when I first heard about the new COX-2 inhibitors, or Super Aspirins, I'll admit I was a bit skeptical. After all, I had treated thousands of arthritis patients for more than two decades and had heard of many "miraculous" cures for arthritis pain—cures that never really panned out in patient trials. Although the primary effect on arthritis symptoms may have been beneficial, the side effects usually added to my patients' worries.

But the Super Aspirins seemed different. As I read study after scientific study on how these compounds actually stop pain without stomach upset, it made sense to me that COX-2 inhibitors were the answer for arthritis sufferers.

To manage arthritis and end the long-term pain, you must first reduce inflammation and stop the inflammatory cycle. Until now, NSAIDs were the trusted medications to slow inflammation. As I've explained, aspirin and NSAIDs block the enzyme *cyclooxygenase,* the enzyme responsible for making prostaglandins—enzymes of inflammation—that subsequently produce pain, swelling, and stiffness in the joints. But NSAIDs block both types of COX enzyme: COX-1 enzymes, which are continuously produced and make prostaglandins that protect the stomach lining and kidneys (and also affect blood platelets); and COX-2 enzymes, which produce the ''bad'' prostaglandins in areas of inflammation.

As I tell my patients, with the COX-2 inhibitors scientists have finally produced a medication that will solve the problem of stomach or intestinal upset because COX-2 inhibitors:

- leave *on* COX-1 enzymes, that are necessary for stomach protection; and

- turn *off* COX-2 enzymes and the subsequent inflammation and pain.

Although these miraculous drugs actually block or inhibit COX-2 enzymes (the ones that produce prostaglandin messengers to cause inflammation, pain, and fever), they do not

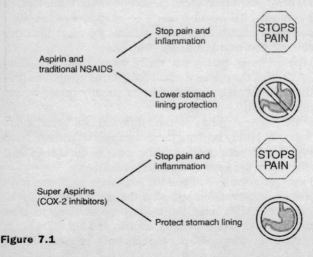

Figure 7.1

block COX-1 enzymes, which are necessary for the health of the stomach.

The Super Aspirin Clinical Trials

Our group has been involved in clinical trials for Super Aspirins and other breakthrough medications for inflammatory arthritis for several years. During this time, the results of our studies on hundreds of adult men and women who have osteoarthritis or rheumatoid arthritis have been combined with the results of studies from across the nation. In study after study the results are the same: ***Super Aspirins stop arthritis pain without side effects.***

If you've had gastrointestinal or other problems taking aspirin or one of the traditional NSAIDs, ask your doctor about the Super Aspirins. We tested some of the Super Aspirins in clinical trials reviewed by the FDA before approval.

THE FIRST SUPER ASPIRINS	
NAME	**DOSAGE**
Celebrex (celecoxib)	Twice a day
Vioxx (rofecoxib)	Once a day
Mobic (meloxicam)	Once a day

In chapter 1, I shared some success stories; here are the results of the clinical trials on the three Super Aspirins in more detail.

Super Aspirins Work for Osteoarthritis

CELEBREX

The Super Aspirin Celebrex (celecoxib) is taken twice daily.

■ In one of the earliest Super Aspirin studies, 300 men and women with osteoarthritis in the knee were given either Celebrex, one of the Super Aspirins, or a placebo. After a fourteen-week period, the Celebrex group reported significantly greater improvement in pain than the control group. Of the patients who took Celebrex, more patients remained in the study because of the excellent pain relief with no serious side effects.

■ In a twelve-week study of more than a thousand men and women with osteoarthritis in the knee, patients whose arthritis was flaring up were given varying doses of Celebrex or naproxen (a traditional NSAID that relieves arthritis pain) or a placebo. All patients took the medication twice daily. Those who took Celebrex at either 100 milligrams or 200 milligrams reported as much pain relief as those who took naproxen, but without stomach upset.

After being diagnosed with osteoarthritis in the hip, forty-seven-year-old Teresa volunteered for a clinical trial, and for months she took Celebrex. She said:

> If you haven't had arthritis, you have no idea what it feels like to hurt all day and all night. My sleep was disrupted every time I rolled over on the arthritic hip in bed. Not only did I feel pain, but I felt exhausted and irritable all the time.
>
> I couldn't take NSAIDs because of a very sensitive stomach, so I relied on acetaminophen, which never gave great relief of pain. In the study I took medicine twice a day. It was like a miracle to me, as after about three weeks I awoke one day and my hip did not hurt. I could hardly believe it but I

sure wasn't going to second-guess a much-needed cure for my pain. Today I am as active as I've ever been—and my mood has changed, too. My family appreciates Celebrex because I'm not short-tempered any longer. It definitely worked for me!

VIOXX

The Super Aspirin Vioxx (rofecoxib) is taken once daily.

■ In another study, 472 volunteers with osteoarthritis took either Vioxx or diclofenac, a well-established, effective NSAID treatment, for more than six months. These men's and women's pain lessened when walking, and their own assessment of their arthritis condition improved. The patients taking Vioxx did as well as those on diclofenac, yet the Super Aspirin had no serious gastrointestinal side effects.

■ In a study of 565 men and women with osteoarthritis volunteers were given either varying doses of Vioxx for six weeks or a placebo. Researchers evaluated the patients' emotional well-being as well as their overall quality of life. Those treated with Vioxx showed improved mental health scores, such as better social functioning and fewer problems with work, as well as significant reductions in pain and improvement in activities of daily living, including eating, bathing, dressing, walking, lifting, bending, working in the house, and participation in sports.

Fifty-year-old Paul felt relief with Vioxx in just four days and was able to start a walking program again with his wife. "The combination of moist heat, exercise, and Vioxx allows me to be as active as I want to," he said. Dorothy, age fifty-nine, felt similarly. She recalled:

Arthritis had stolen my life. I used to be so active and played golf every weekend with my husband. But in the past four years, I've done nothing but sit on my porch and watch others. Within two weeks on

Vioxx, my osteoarthritis pain in the hips and knees had decreased so much that I could hardly believe it. By the study's third week, I could walk up the steps to my porch without any pain or stiffness. I knew then that I could also play golf. Ray, my husband, and I started with nine holes of golf the next Saturday, and I loved every minute of it. I used moist heat applications after the golf game, as well as with my morning shower, and I think this helped keep me flexible.

MOBIC

Mobic (meloxicam) is another Super Aspirin that is already approved for use in many countries. It is taken once daily.

■ In a clinical trial using Mobic on men and women with osteoarthritis in the knee, researchers tracked the joint pain in 513 osteoarthritis patients and found that Mobic was more effective in controlling osteoarthritis symptoms and as well tolerated as the placebo or inactive medicine. Volunteers who took Mobic reported pain levels dropping significantly during the first two weeks. If these volunteers had taken a traditional NSAID in the amounts necessary to feel such a decrease in pain, the chances of gastrointestinal problems would be higher.

■ A study of 455 patients with osteoarthritis in the knee or hip who were treated with Mobic reported improvement similar to that from Feldene (piroxicam), yet the Super Aspirin was well tolerated without significant side effects. Feldene is an established arthritis drug.

■ Another analysis of more than 5,500 patients from a number of countries showed Mobic was better tolerated than commonly prescribed NSAIDs with no loss of ability to relieve pain and inflammation. In one study the number of hospital stays was 95 percent lower in the patients who took Mobic, because of fewer peptic ulcer complications. These patients also reported lower pain scores on Mobic. Some studies showed as much as an 85 percent reduction in peptic ulcers, intestinal bleeding, and intestinal perforation (which usually requires an operation). Gastrointestinal side effects were less common in the Mobic patients; in fact, the gastrointestinal side effects of Mobic were comparable to that of the placebo. Mobic has been shown to have no deleterious effect on kidney function or platelets when given at the 7.5 mg daily dose. Studies showed that both 7.5 mg and 15 mg of Mobic once daily worked, and both doses were comparable to piroxicam (Feldene), diclofenac (Voltaren), and naproxen (Naprosyn) (all effective arthritis treatments listed in chapter 6).

Fifty-four-year-old Carole, who had osteoarthritis in the hip, was unable to take traditional NSAIDs because of chronic stomach problems. She volunteered for a Super Aspirin study and took Mobic once a day. In less than six days, Carole felt a dramatic reduction in pain and less fatigue because she could finally sleep without hip pain. "For years I would wake up at least every hour because my hip would ache when I rolled over in bed. After just six days on Mobic, I slept through the night with no hip pain."

Super Aspirins and Rheumatoid Arthritis

Realizing that Super Aspirins could help those with osteoarthritis, researchers decided to investigate whether COX-2 inhibitors could help those with rheumatoid arthritis.

- Clinical trials on 1,100 rheumatoid arthritis patients revealed that those who received Celebrex had decreased pain and swelling in their joints, as did those who received naproxen, but those on Celebrex didn't suffer from the stomach upset associated with naproxen.

■ In another trial of over 300 men and women with rheumatoid arthritis, half were given Celebrex; half took the placebo in place of their usual treatments. Again, significantly fewer patients who took Celebrex dropped out of the clinical trial because their arthritis pain and stiffness worsened. This exciting study revealed Celebrex does work to stop pain and inflammation in rheumatoid arthritis. The minimal side effects on those treated with Celebrex were no more than on those who took a placebo. This is important, because many medications for rheumatoid arthritis have serious side effects.

Catherine found that Celebrex gave her so much relief for rheumatoid arthritis pain that she was able to go back to work part-time. This thirty-nine-year-old attorney had taken a leave of absence from practicing law. She said:

In less than two weeks, the overall pain had decreased greatly. I'll never forget the day I got out of bed, and I could put my weight on my feet and I didn't wince in pain. It gave me hope that I could be active again and even motivated me to be more consistent with the twice-daily exercises and applications of moist heat. I had been reluctant to do these for several months because when I moved around more, it hurt! Now I'm able to exercise all my joints in full range of motion and work afternoons at my law firm.

Other volunteers had similar stories of reduced pain and stiffness:

■ Maria, forty-four, began a walking program just two weeks into the Celebrex trial for rheumatoid arthritis and experienced an increase in energy because of less pain and sounder sleep.

- John, thirty-seven, was more productive at work because he didn't feel the gnawing stomach pains caused by traditional NSAIDs.

- Stanley, sixty-two, who had taken early retirement because of severe pain caused by rheumatoid arthritis, began to volunteer at a nearby hospital, helping children with arthritis.

- Karen, forty-nine, found that she had more mobility in her hands and greatly reduced pain. She was able to play the piano again at her church after not playing for more than three years.

All Types of Arthritis

Although these COX-2 inhibitors have been tested mainly on osteoarthritis and rheumatoid arthritis patients, many scientists believe they will benefit other conditions such as fibromyalgia, bursitis, tendinitis, and psoriatic arthritis, among many. Some patients with other less common types of arthritis such as ankylosing spondylitis have taken Super Aspirins with good results.

Super Aspirins Are Safe to Use

As demonstrated by the studies described above, Super Aspirins relieve pain without stomach side effects. The most common side effects reported so far with the new Super Aspirins are diarrhea, headache, and insomnia—but these side effects were also found in patients taking the placebo.

To validate the claim that the Super Aspirins didn't cause stomach complications, scientists, in a safety study, compared Super Aspirins to traditional NSAIDs and other medications, as well as to placebos. Healthy patients (those without arthritis or other diseases) were given Celebrex twice daily and reported no more peptic ulcers than those who took no medicine at all. Patients taking naproxen (a traditional

NSAID for treating arthritis) were found to have a higher rate of gastric ulcers.

What we noticed in our Super Aspirin clinical trials was that fewer patients dropped out because they didn't find relief of arthritis pain. With Super Aspirins, patients who have not taken their traditional arthritis medication because of stomach upset can now comply with doctors' recommendations. As one patient involved in the clinical trials said, "I used to get the prescription for the NSAID filled but wouldn't even open the bottle because I knew my stomach would ache all day. When I was on the Super Aspirins study, I took the medication without fear of side effects and was able to be active again."

Keep in mind that the Super Aspirins have not been tested on children or pregnant women, so they should not be taken in these situations unless your doctor has advised you. And Super Aspirins will not duplicate the effect of regular aspirin taken daily to lower the chance of blood clots or heart attacks because they don't affect platelets.

Super Aspirins May Prevent Cancer and Other Diseases

Early studies indicate that COX-2 inhibitors may do much more than relieve arthritis pain and stiffness: Super Aspirins may prevent colon cancer, Alzheimer's disease, and osteoporosis (thinning of the bones). Although these are all preliminary studies, they do suggest a potential benefit from the new Super Aspirins.

Colon Cancer

Colon cancer is the second leading cause of cancer death if you count men and women together, and the American Cancer Society predicts that more than 95,000 Americans will die of colon cancer this year. Researchers are finding a link between COX-2 and colon cancer, and many speculate that by blocking COX-2, Super Aspirins may help to prevent this deadly disease.

Since 1991, studies of arthritis patients who took aspirin or traditional NSAIDs on a regular basis consistently indicate a lower risk of colon cancer. In a group of arthritis patients in 1996, researchers discovered 45 percent fewer deaths from colon cancer. Why? Scientists theorized that aspirin and traditional NSAIDs prevented the growth of tumor cells, thus lowering the chances of colon cancer.

Vanderbilt University researchers found high levels of COX-2 in 90 percent of colon tumors. These same researchers found that COX-2 was not only present in higher amounts in colon cancers but that some cells were much ''less susceptible to death.'' Programmed death is the usual way abnormal cells are eliminated from the body, so when cells are less susceptible to death, abnormal cancer cells are not eliminated as easily and could stick around to cause future cancers.

Other researchers have reported that when mice who usually develop cancer were given Celebrex, the development of tumors was reduced by two-thirds. One group of researchers treated rats with chemicals that increase the incidence of colon cancers. One group was given a diet including Celebrex while the other group's diet contained no Celebrex. The Celebrex group had a 93 percent reduced incidence of colon tumors and this effect on colon tumors was more pronounced than that of other traditional NSAIDs from previous experiments. So Celebrex could prevent colon tumors in rats. Still other scientists found that when mice who usually develop cancer were given Celebrex, the development of tumors was reduced by two-thirds.

Studies are now being done to see if colon cancer might be prevented in humans who are at higher risk for this disease. Some research already suggests that NSAIDs can prevent colon tumors in families who have a higher risk of cancer. Although the cancer–COX-2 inhibitor link is still not fully understood, researchers believe that definitive answers are just a few years away.

Alzheimer's Disease

While studying the COX-2 inhibitors as treatment for pain and inflammation, scientists realized another unexpected positive effect. Fascinating studies from Mount Sinai Medical Center in New York reported finding twice as much COX-2 in brains of Alzheimer's patients as in healthy persons.

Scientists speculate that the higher enzyme level may contribute to the formation of a protein plaque that kills brain cells. Although the exact connection has not yet been identified, this finding is exciting. Other researchers have found a much-reduced incidence of Alzheimer's disease in people who regularly take aspirin or traditional NSAIDs. This crucial issue is now being investigated as another possible benefit of COX-2 inhibitors.

Kidney Disease

Not surprisingly, COX-2 inhibitors work in other ways that may be important to your health. By not interfering with COX-1 enzymes, they allow the regulation of the kidney function to continue normally. This can be important for those who develop kidney problems from traditional NSAIDs. Although kidney complications in NSAID patients are not very common (less than 1 percent develop a problem), they can be very serious when they happen.

Researchers have found that COX-2 may influence blood flow in kidneys and could play a role in chronic kidney disease. In laboratory studies, when COX-2 enzyme was blocked in rats, scientists realized there was also less kidney damage. This early finding shows more exciting promise for the Super Aspirins.

Osteoporosis

At the University of Connecticut, researchers found a possible link between COX-2 enzymes and osteoporosis in mice.

If COX-2 enzymes are in fact important in osteoporosis, COX-2 inhibitors may offer some protection. More studies are now beginning to answer this question.

Menstrual Cramps

For women, COX-2 inhibitors may solve an ongoing problem that most medications cannot. In clinical trials, women who suffered from painful menstrual cramps found relief with COX-2 inhibitors. In some studies, Vioxx gave relief comparable to ibuprofen and placebo, but without any stomach upset. Some volunteers, such as Erin, found that the Super Aspirins gave better relief for cramps than ibuprofen. She said:

> I used to play college basketball, and a knee injury caused me to get OA at age thirty-two, so I volunteered for the Super Aspirin study for osteoarthritis of the knees. I took Vioxx once a day, and in about ten days my knee virtually quit aching. It was super to be able to walk and move around without waiting for intense pain to jolt up my thigh and remind me of this horrible problem. Yet I also received an added benefit—a great reduction in menstrual cramping. I've always had horrible PMS, with cramps that hurt worse than giving birth! I had been on Vioxx for three weeks when I realized that my period was about to start and I had no cramps as a warning sign. This was more than I had hoped for when I signed up for the trial, but I'll be first in line for a prescription when Super Aspirins hit the market.

Will Super Aspirins Work for You?

"These studies and testimonials are great. But will they work for me?" That's what most patients ask when they hear about something as amazing as the Super Aspirins. A good way to evaluate how the Super Aspirins control your arthritis pain is to chart your "pain" days when you start taking one of the new Super Aspirins. Use the following calendar and circle the days when your arthritis pain is immobilizing or keeps you from your daily activities.

PAIN CALENDAR						
1	2	3	4	5	6	7
8	9	10	11	12	13	14
15	16	17	18	19	20	21
22	23	24	25	26	27	28

During this time, also start the specific arthritis treatment your doctor prescribes or use the treatment plan outlined in chapter 9—don't skip one step of moist heat applications and exercise! Review this calendar in four weeks. If you circled more days than not, or if the pain is not reduced or has increased, this may indicate that the Super Aspirin did not work well in your situation. Ask your doctor to try another Super Aspirin or another new medication to help end your pain and stiffness.

Of course, as with any medication, not everyone who takes the Super Aspirins improves. Your doctor can help you decide which medication would be worthwhile to try.

The Future of Pain Relief

For our rapidly aging nation, Super Aspirins promise to change the way we live. They reduce the joint pain and inflammation caused by arthritis and relieve the pain of other health problems—without side effects on the kidneys or stomach. And COX-2 inhibitors may even protect us from colon cancer, Alzheimer's disease, and kidney disease. These "wonder drugs" may become just as common as a daily vitamin tablet for millions of people.

....

CHAPTER 8

More Breakthrough Arthritis Treatments

The Super Aspirins promise to change the way those with arthritis live, offering relief of pain and stiffness without stomach problems. However, there are a host of other breakthrough treatments that I believe will offer great benefits for rheumatoid arthritis sufferers. At Tampa Medical Group Research, we have done clinical trials on many of these new arthritis drugs. Some have been released, while others are being developed for the approval of the Food and Drug Administration (FDA) specifically for use in arthritis.

As I explain in this chapter, the medications include new biologic response modifiers. Biologic treatments affect the specific cells that cause inflammation, pain, swelling, and destruction in arthritis, or they affect the products these cells make, which then create inflammation. Although tumor necrosis factor (TNF), a protein made of amino acids, is one of the most important products of the cells that create inflammation, there are also others. Some of the new treatments now available can slow or stop TNF—and stop pain and swelling dramatically. Some attack the cells that make the inflammation-causing enzymes; others interrupt the messages of inflammation by stopping the abnormal cells from making contact with other cells.

Another way to stop abnormal cells from causing inflammation is to stop the chemical messengers they produce. These chemical messengers actually trigger the reactions that cause pain, swelling, and stiffness in joints. By stopping these chemicals, the inflammation and destruction may be stopped as well.

Stopping Rheumatoid Arthritis in Its Tracks

As explained in chapter 4, rheumatoid arthritis (RA) occurs when your immune system goes haywire and attacks your joints, unlike osteoarthritis, which results from the wear and tear of joints. As the immune cells and their products eat away at your cartilage and eventually erode your bones, your RA could become crippling. The good news is that the new medications may prevent or halt this damage.

In RA, TNF is overproduced in the joints. Researchers believe that TNF may be responsible for directing destruction of bone and cartilage. TNF can also cause pain, fever, weight loss, and the fatigue associated with rheumatoid arthritis. Understanding that TNF may trigger many other enzymes, scientists now conclude that blocking TNF should greatly relieve the effects of inflammation. There are several different types of new drugs that block TNF.

Much of the future success of these breakthrough medicines for rheumatoid arthritis depends on early diagnosis and treatment before there is permanent bone and joint destruction. In the past, arthritis specialists waited until rheumatoid arthritis was well established to begin treatment with medicines, such as gold, methotrexate, azathioprine, cyclophosphamide, and cyclosporine (explained later in this chapter), intended to slow or stop the course of the arthritis. Permanent changes in the joints were often already apparent. One reason they waited to treat was their concern over the grave side effects of these medicines involving the kidney, the liver, and the blood.

When rheumatoid arthritis is far enough along to cause

permanent changes in the joints, the destruction is irreversible. Once specialists realized that much destruction occurs early in rheumatoid arthritis, they become more willing to use the ''stronger'' medicines early to try to stop the arthritis before it takes hold.

Comprehensive research now confirms that aggressive treatment using stronger drugs within the first year of diagnosing rheumatoid arthritis often gives better results than just using NSAIDs. Delaying a diagnosis and its subsequent treatment may hurt you eventually, especially once joint destruction begins.

The following breakthrough treatments offer good results for control of rheumatoid arthritis with few serious side effects. Because FDA approval is pending for some of these medicines ask your doctor which one is available to help you.

Enbrel

Enbrel (etanercept) is a genetically engineered medication that works by soaking up excess TNF, thus breaking the chain of events that causes inflammation, pain, swelling, and joint damage. In clinical trials, Enbrel has been studied in more than one thousand rheumatoid arthritis patients. In one study, 180 rheumatoid arthritis patients who had not responded to other standard treatments took Enbrel injections for three months. The under-the-skin injections, like insulin shots, are given two times weekly in 25-milligram doses. Researchers concluded that joint pain and swelling decreased with Enbrel after assessing laboratory tests and physicians' and patients' descriptions of their conditions and overall quality of life.

Seventy-five percent of the patients who received Enbrel reported more than 20 percent improvement in symptoms, while only 14 percent of other patients improved. The Enbrel volunteers reported a 61 percent reduction in the number of swollen and tender joints, while patients on the placebo reported only 25 percent. Pain and morning stiffness decreased and quality of life improved. The side effects of Enbrel were few, including mild reactions at the injection site and symptoms of mild upper-respiratory infections (colds, cough, runny nose, or sinusitis); researchers found no kidney, liver, or blood problems as side effects.

In another study of patients who took Enbrel for six months, roughly the same percentage (75 percent) felt a decrease in joint pain, stiffness, and swelling. In some cases, patients noticed improvement within four to eight weeks of starting treatment. Patients reported as much as 69 percent reduction in their estimation of pain. And in long-term trials, 59 percent of patients in the study maintained a good response for six months. In some cases, improvement has lasted longer than eighteen months.

Lynn, a thirty-seven-year-old editor, had suffered from rheumatoid arthritis for a decade when she volunteered for her trial. She had difficulty typing on the computer because of pain and stiffness in her hands and wrist. Yet after three weeks on the medication, Lynn's pain level dramatically decreased, making it easier for her to work on her computer as well as exercise. Lynn's success with Enbrel is consistent with thousands of others who participated in clinical trials. Overall, the results of studies on Enbrel appear extremely hopeful and promising. If the results continue to show improvement in joint pain and swelling with prevention of joint damage, the lack of side effects may make Enbrel a major improvement in the treatment of rheumatoid arthritis.

Enbrel, approved by the FDA, is intended for those patients with moderate to severe rheumatoid arthritis who have not responded adequately to other medications, such as the slow-acting medicines on pages 93–98. Enbrel may be combined with methotrexate if your arthritis specialist feels this is necessary. If you develop a serious infection you should stop Enbrel.

Since Enbrel is given by injection, you should take the first shot in your doctor's office, or a nurse should be present to be sure it is given correctly. Because the medicine must be mixed with the sterile water supplied in the package, be sure your doctor or nurse shows you how to mix it properly. An instruction sheet is provided.

Enbrel is expensive to produce, so it will cost more than most medicines used today for rheumatoid arthritis. Still, if it prevents progression of the disease, it will be an excellent value because it has fewer side effects. There is no evidence so far that Enbrel makes one vulnerable to life-threatening diseases, although this is still being studied. The savings in expense from preventing disability; other chronic treatment costs; and the costs of side effects, hospitalization, and surgeries will increase the value of treatments such as Enbrel.

Remicade

Remicade (infliximab) is an antibody specifically designed to find TNF and neutralize it. This medication is given by intravenous injection.

In one study, about 60 percent of rheumatoid arthritis patients improved when they were treated with Remicade weekly for fourteen weeks. When Remicade was given in combination with methotrexate, an older drug used for rheumatoid arthritis (described on page 94), researchers found 70 to 90 percent improvement in joint pain and swelling that lasted for twenty-six weeks in many patients. In 428 patients with rheumatoid arthritis, Remicade reduced swollen joints by 57 percent in patients who took Remicade compared with placebo. Twenty-eight percent of those treated with Remicade achieved a 50 percent reduction in symptoms at 30 weeks compared with only 5 percent of those on placebo. Most patients who responded to Remicade could tell a difference within the first two weeks of treatment, up to six weeks.

The most common side effects were upper respiratory tract infections, headache, nausea, sinusitis, rash, and cough.

Remicade is also used to treat Crohn's disease, inflammation of the intestine, which causes diarrhea and abdominal pain.

Arava

Arava (leflunomide), another breakthrough treatment specifically developed for rheumatoid arthritis in the past decade,
works by blocking an enzyme called *dihydroorotate
dehydrogenase* (DHODH). This slows down the lymphocytes, white blood cells that trigger inflammation involved in
the process that leads to RA, and subsequently slows the
progression of the disease.

In clinical trials, researchers measured improvement of
rheumatoid arthritis patients by taking x-rays of hands and
feet at the start of the study, then tracked these people
throughout the entire period. In clinical studies of 480 patients with rheumatoid arthritis, researchers found that after
one year, those taking Arava showed four times less deterio-
ration in the x-rays than those taking the placebo. Arava
slowed the progression of RA more than methotrexate, a
traditional RA drug. In another study of 402 rheumatoid
patients, almost 60 percent responded with reduced pain and
swelling in their joints. It may take as long as one to two
months for Arava's benefits to be noticed, but you may continue to see improvement for five to six months.

Of the patients who took Arava during the clinical trials,
the most commonly reported side effects (one-fourth or
more) were diarrhea, rash, and hair loss. Researchers found
that Arava can take six months or more to clear the body and
can cause birth defects in animals. Women who are or might
become pregnant should not take Arava. Men should not take
Arava if there is a chance they might conceive a child while
taking Arava.

The FDA advises women or men who have used Arava
and might become pregnant to take cholestyramine, a medication that helps eliminate Arava more quickly from the
blood. Tests should be done to be sure Arava is eliminated
before any pregnancy commences. Your doctor can guide
you. Regular blood tests are also needed to check for liver
abnormalities or other abnormal lab results.

AnervaX

AnervaX, a new injectable medication, is the first vaccine ever developed specifically for rheumatoid arthritis. The idea of a vaccine is not new, but only lately has there been a drug that shows a positive response in patients with severe rheumatoid arthritis. AnervaX blocks the work of the T cell, the lymphocyte known to play a role in causing rheumatoid arthritis pain, swelling, and stiffness. Further clinical trials of the vaccine are now in progress although initial small studies show improvement. Ask your arthritis specialist to keep you posted as the trial results become known.

Prosorba Column

Prosorba uses a special column through which blood is treated in a machine (column) by apheresis, a technique in which blood is removed, treated, and then returned to the donor. Blood is drawn similar to the method used during blood donation. With a prosorba column, the patient's blood is removed from a vein in an arm by a needle and treated as it passes through the column. During this process, certain proteins in the blood that lead to inflammation are removed, and the blood is returned to your body.

This treatment is for severe cases of rheumatoid arthritis that do not respond to other treatment. In clinical trials, no serious side effects have been reported. Of ninety-one patients, 45 percent improved, while only 13.3 percent of the placebo treatments responded. The treatment effect can be long-lasting, with some patients able to stay off treatment for as long as seventy-five weeks. The average duration of the response was about forty weeks.

Colloral

Colloral—a medication made from chicken cartilage—is a new treatment for rheumatoid arthritis, even though it has been studied in animals and humans for other problems in the past. It was first used in clinical trials with the rationale that because cartilage may be a main target of the antibodies that trigger the pain and swelling, giving small doses of the very substance that the body is fighting might build up the body's immunity to it.

Some earlier studies showed slight improvement in rheumatoid arthritis patients treated with colloral, but not a dramatic response. In a trial with 274 patients treated for six months, some patients improved but it wasn't a measurable, statistically significant response. Still, more than half of the patients reported some improvement in joint pain and swelling. And some treated with colloral even maintained their improvement after the treatment ended. More testing needs to be done to determine the best dose, as well as when this treatment is most effective.

What's appealing is the apparent lack of side effects, but nonetheless, I'm concerned about remedies sold at local health food stores that claim to contain cartilage as an arthritis treatment. As with all unapproved medications, unless you are participating in a clinical trial, you should be suspicious of unknown drugs because problems could arise from impure products that contain other substances, and the side effects from large doses or even small doses over a long period of time are not known.

Current Slow-Acting Drugs for Rheumatoid Arthritis

The slow-acting or disease-modifying medicines are added when rheumatoid arthritis pain and swelling remain a problem even after using moist heat, exercises, and Super Aspirins or traditional NSAIDs. These medications work slowly and control or suppress the arthritis at a more basic level. Because they are less expensive and arthritis specialists have more experience using these medications, they are recommended first before the breakthrough medicines already discussed.

In the past, the slow-acting medications were not used until after deformities developed—often years after the rheumatoid arthritis started. Now we know that the best results may happen when they are started during the first year or so of the rheumatoid arthritis. This is when it is apparent that the arthritis is out of control or at least as soon as permanent changes are visible on x-rays. If one or more of these drugs does not make your rheumatoid arthritis livable, your arthritis specialist will probably consider one of the newer breakthrough medicines.

Methotrexate

Methotrexate (Rheumatrex tablets and injectable methotrexate) is the most popular of the slow-acting medicines used to try to stop the progress of rheumatoid arthritis. More than 80 percent of rheumatoid patients respond with reduced pain and swelling. In some cases it may completely control the RA symptoms. It may also delay the progress of bone destruction.

Methotrexate may be combined with other traditional NSAIDs for a better effect. The most common side effect is nausea, which usually occurs within one day of taking the weekly dose of methotrexate. If the nausea is too bothersome, the methotrexate may be given by injection in a muscle, which can diminish the nausea. Mild side effects, such as mouth sores, may be controlled by taking a folic acid supplement. Abnormal liver tests, abnormal blood counts (red cells, white cells, platelet counts), and lung reactions such as pneumonia are uncommon but can occur, so regular blood tests and checkups are important.

Azulfidine

Azulfidine (sulfasalazine) is another slow-acting medicine used to treat rheumatoid arthritis that does not respond to anti-inflammatory drugs. This tablet is usually well tolerated and has about a 70 percent chance of decreasing joint pain

nd stiffness. The improvement may begin four to twelve
veeks after starting the medicine. Some studies show it may
low the progress of arthritis.

The most common side effects are usually mild and in-
:lude loss of appetite, headache, nausea, vomiting, and upset
tomach. Azulfidine occasionally causes abnormal blood and
iver tests, including anemia, low white blood cell count, or
•ther blood abnormality. If you try Azulfidine, your doctor
vill schedule you for regular blood tests.

Plaquenil

•laquenil (hydroxychloroquine) may be the slow-acting med-
cation with the fewest side effects. The tablet can relieve
oint pain and stiffness, and may be used along with other
nedications such as an NSAID or combined with methotrex-
ite to improve the effect. You'll need to have an eye examina-
ion once or twice each year to watch for side effects in your
etina, which are actually extremely rare.

Gold Capsules and Injections

Gold medications have been used for many years, because
hey effectively relieve symptoms and may slow or stop the
lestructive progress of rheumatoid arthritis. The capsules
Ridaura) are convenient but have a lower response rate than
;old injections. The most common side effect of Ridaura is
liarrhea, which affects 30 percent of patients but then often
eases without stopping the medications.

Gold injections (Myochrisine, Solganal) are given in the
iip muscle and are usually tolerated well. About 70 to 75
•ercent of patients respond with decreased pain and swelling.
The most common side effects are rash or mouth sores. Reg-
lar blood counts and urinalysis are needed with all gold
nedications to check for side effects on the bone marrow and
:idneys.

Imuran

Imuran (azathioprine) is an effective medicine for rheumatoid arthritis and is also used to treat other diseases, including cancer. The response rate is as good as to methotrexate and gold, and patients may stay on this medication for long periods of time. The side effects are usually mild, with occasional nausea. Regular blood counts are needed to check for safety and for the effects of Imuran on the bone marrow.

Minocycline

The antibiotic Minocycline may benefit those with rheumatoid arthritis. When researchers erroneously thought that rheumatoid arthritis was caused by infection (especially in cases when it came on suddenly or followed what seemed to be an infection), they thought the antibiotic might help by curing the underlying infection.

Nevertheless, Minocycline may help arthritis in other ways, possibly acting as an anti-inflammatory drug. In one trial of eighty patients, 38 percent had a decrease in pain and swelling compared with 18 percent of placebo patients. In another study 65 percent of patients treated with Minocycline improved compared with 13 percent of placebo patients. Side effects were usually mild, with gastrointestinal symptoms and dizziness most commonly reported.

Overall, Minocycline seems safe and, although not a dramatic breakthrough, it may give relief to some patients.

Cyclosporine and Neoral

Cyclosporine and its newer form, Neoral, are used to treat severe cases of rheumatoid arthritis that do not respond to any other available medicines discussed so far. These strong medicines may have serious side effects, especially on the kidneys. Cyclosporine attacks the lymphocytes that direct the inflammatory process, especially the ones that are active in rheumatoid arthritis. (Renal transplant patients take it to prevent rejection of the transplant by the patient's immune system.)

Neoral, the newer form of cyclosporine, is a special preparation that may act more predictably in the body. Overall, cyclosporine, especially Neoral, can offer relief to many patients with severe rheumatoid arthritis, especially those who have not responded to other medications. The improvement usually begins in four to eight weeks. Neoral is combined with methotrexate in some cases to control more severe rheumatoid arthritis. Your doctor or arthritis specialist must monitor you closely so that side effects can be avoided; the most common are kidney problems; hypertension; headache; gastrointestinal problems such as nausea, indigestion, diarrhea, or abdominal pain; and increased hair growth. Your doctor will watch closely for changes in blood pressure, using blood tests to ensure there are no side effects on the kidneys, liver, or other functions.

Cytoxan and Leukeran

Cytoxan (cyclophosphamide) and Leukeran (chlorambucil) are two effective medicines for rheumatoid arthritis that effectively relieve pain and swelling in severe cases. However, the benefits do not usually outweigh the risks. These include effects on the bone marrow, blood in the urine from bladder infection, hair loss, and increased cancer risk, when these drugs are taken over a period of a few years. These drugs are not used very often by arthritis specialists.

Cuprimine

Cuprimine (penicillamine), taken as a capsule, must be administered for several months before its effectiveness can be measured in a particular case of rheumatoid arthritis. Because it takes so long to work and the chances of response are only moderate, it is used infrequently by arthritis specialists. Cuprimine is usually tolerated by patients, but regular blood

counts and urine tests are needed to monitor side effects on
the bone marrow and kidneys.

Creams and Rubs

Some creams have been found to give temporary relief for
arthritis. Capsaicin cream (Zostrix and other brands), available over the counter at most drug or grocery stores, probably
has been studied the most. Made from chili peppers, it warms
the skin when it is applied over the joint. It may slow down
the chemicals produced by the body that send pain messages
from the joint. It's safe to try, although some feel it makes
their skin feel uncomfortably hot. Follow the package directions for best results.

Creams that contain NSAIDs have been available in other
countries for years and are now becoming popular in the
United States. NSAID creams deliver the medication directly
to the site, which may avoid most of the side effects of taking
NSAIDs orally. To use the cream, apply a small amount over
the joint, two or three times daily. Only a small percentage of
the drug is absorbed into your system, so side effects are not
very common.

Talk with your doctor before you use any of these creams.
Diclofenac, naproxen, ibuprofen, piroxicam, and other
NSAIDs can be made into a treatment cream by your phar-
macist, but you will need a prescription from your doctor.

Injections to End Osteoarthritis Pain

Hyalgan, Synvisc, and Orthovisc (hyaluronic acid) are new
treatments for osteoarthritis that are given by injection directly into the knee. These medications differ from corticosteroid drugs used for many years in many kinds of
arthritis.

Hyaluronic acid is a part of normal joint fluid and helps
make the fluid more elastic and protective of the cartilage

surface in the joint, which has become worn in osteoarthritis. Injected as a medicine, hyaluronic acid can relieve pain and stiffness.

Studies of my patients using these injections have shown decreased pain and a possible added effect of reduced breakdown of the knee cartilage. In one study, injectable Synvisc relieved pain and improved function, with fewer side effects than daily traditional NSAID treatments, over twelve weeks. Several patients have used these injections after other medicines gave no improvement, especially when they were considering surgery. The results were very promising:

- A fifty-five-year-old restaurant owner stopped using a cane, which he had used for several months because of pain.

- A sixty-year-old secretary found she could do almost all of her activities at work without pain.

- A fifty-nine-year-old homemaker was able to take care of her family with fewer rest periods during the day.

If you try an injectable medication for OA, it's important to keep up your usual moist heat, exercises, and Super Aspirin or other NSAID just as you would with other treatments. Unfortunately, if your knees are so badly worn that you no longer have any cartilage, the injections probably won't work.

One advantage of injecting hyaluronic acid is that it is not a corticosteroid drug and does not go throughout the entire body but is targeted only at the knee. Also, the positive effects of the injection on joint pain and stiffness last longer than most corticosteroid injections. In clinical trials, 65 to 80 percent of those who received these injections reported reduced pain and stiffness; improvement lasted five to seven months.

The injections (a total of three to five given weekly) are more expensive than cortisone shots, but the lack of side effects and the possibility of prolonged response make this a good choice if other treatments do not work or you cannot take them. This treatment is not recommended if there is bone rubbing against bone in the knee due to the loss of cartilage. These injections are not used for rheumatoid arthritis. Your doctor can guide you.

Estrogen

Can estrogen, the major female hormone, prevent or treat arthritis? In women with osteoarthritis, symptoms often worsen after menopause, when estrogen levels drop. This raises the possibility that estrogen might help prevent osteoarthritis or protect cartilage.

There has been no definite proof yet, but women who take estrogen after menopause often have fewer complaints of osteoarthritis. Some intriguing studies are being done now in England on the estrogen-OA link. In one study of more than six hundred women, scientists found that those who took estrogen had less chance of developing osteoarthritis in their knees.

So far, there is not enough evidence to warrant treating osteoarthritis with estrogen. When estrogen was used in the past to treat other types of arthritis, such as rheumatoid arthritis, it was not proven to reduce the pain and stiffness.

Managing Your Pain

In our clinics we see rheumatoid arthritis patients who are able to greatly improve their management of pain, inflammation, and stiffness using a combination of medicines, applications of moist heat twice daily, and exercise. Chapter 9 outlines this 5-step program that has helped thousands of our arthritis patients turn their lives around, ending the cycle of pain that has dominated them for years. If you make a personal commitment to finding the most effective medicine for rheumatoid arthritis and diligently follow the steps in the treatment plan, it will help you as well.

CHAPTER **9**

....

5 Steps to
Pain-Free Living

You are taking your first step to pain-free living by using a
Super Aspirin or another of the new arthritis medications.
But there are more steps you can take to manage your arthritis symptoms. I tell all my patients that the best way to
optimize pain control is to follow the five simple steps I
outline in this chapter. By using moist heat, exercising, following a proper diet, and avoiding known arthritis triggers in
conjunction with taking your medications, you can further
minimize your arthritis inflammation and thus reduce your
pain. I urge everyone to incorporate these steps into their
daily routines. Here are the stories of some of my patients
who followed my advice.

Babs was fifty-four when I diagnosed her with osteoarthritis in the shoulder and fibromyalgia. She told me she was an
avid tennis player in her twenties and thirties, but when the
pain and fatigue kicked in, she could hardly swing a racket,
much less brush her hair. Even washing dishes triggered her
pain. Babs tried NSAIDs, but with her history of stomach
problems she couldn't take the medication without feeling
pain and nausea. She thought she'd just "grin and bear the
body that hurts all over," but when she found that she

couldn't hold her baby grandson, she sought new treatment to end her discomfort.

Babs volunteered for a Celebrex clinical trial specifically for osteoarthritis. Along with the medication, she began using moist heat twice a day. She also stretched daily, using range-of-motion exercises to strengthen the muscles that support her shoulder joint. In less than six months while rigorously following the daily treatment program, Babs was virtually pain free. Not only did the osteoarthritis pain subside, but her deep muscle pain of fibromyalgia also eased. She rejoined her tennis team and now baby-sits for her grandson on the weekends.

David's story is typical of many men with osteoarthritis who think that if they ignore it, it will go away. This thirty-eight-year-old professional guitarist came to our clinic because of severe knee pain. He said he had suffered from this pain and stiffness for years after a motorcycle injury in college. He took up to ten over-the-counter NSAIDs every day but quit when he began to feel a gnawing, burning pain in his stomach. And when he couldn't put weight on his leg as he got out of his car, he realized he needed more effective treatment.

After a series of tests, he signed up for the Vioxx clinical trial, then started his own treatment regimen: moist heat twice daily, using a warm shower or a whirlpool bath; swimming laps each day at a neighbor's pool to increase flexibility and strength in his knees; and watching his diet to shed ten pounds.

It took almost four weeks before David admitted that the treatment plan was reducing his pain. And after three months, David experienced an 80 percent improvement of his knee pain; within six months, he felt pain only on the days he ignored his exercises. David was thrilled.

Because arthritis can sometimes be difficult to manage, it may take a few weeks before you notice improvement—remember, it took David almost a month before he felt better. I know it's easy to give up during that time, thinking that nothing can help you. But please don't. Stick with the 5-step plan even if you do not feel immediate results, and in at least one month you will—you'll have less pain and more mobility.

Start with Positive Thinking

No matter how severe your arthritis symptoms are, perhaps the most important factor in gaining control over them is a positive attitude. I make clear to all my patients that if they fight their arthritis with this 5-step treatment program *and* an optimistic and positive attitude, they'll see even better results. Having a positive attitude alone may make the difference between being active each day or having a sedentary life. I have seen patients who were almost crippled by arthritis return to normal activity because they firmly believed the prescribed 5-step program would work. Belief is crucial in overcoming obstacles in life!

The following steps *do work,* so I urge you to follow these easy suggestions. The more committed you are to doing this routine each day, the more long-term relief you will feel.

Step 1: Use Moist Heat Twice Daily

No matter which type of arthritis you have, I recommend twice daily applications of moist heat as a vital part of treatment and pain control. It's simple and inexpensive to do, with great benefits. I've found that in almost all of my patients moist heat makes it easier to exercise aching arthritic joints. You'll get pain relief, relaxed muscles, and increased joint flexibility.

Select the most convenient and beneficial type of moist heat that will help your arthritis:

- Warm shower
- Warm bathtub
- Heated pool
- Hot tub or Jacuzzi

- Warm, moist towels
- Moist heating pad
- Hydrocollator packs
- Paraffin–mineral oil therapeutic mixture for the hands or feet
- Hot water bottle with damp cloth

Use this application *twice every day, without fail.* Start with ten to fifteen minutes each morning and evening. You may have to get up a few minutes earlier in the morning before work, and then make time to do this before bedtime, but this extra time is worth the reduced pain and stiffness you will experience.

After three to four weeks, you may find that your pain has lessened dramatically. Decrease the treatment to one application of moist heat each day. Then, as your levels of pain, swelling, and stiffness improve even more, use the moist heat only when you feel it is needed.

A ten- to fifteen-minute warm shower can give excellent pain relief and help you get through the day without stiffness.

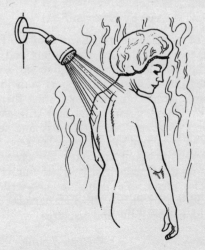

Figure 9.1

The Icing Alternative

Some people prefer to use ice to stop pain and apply ice packs to their joints or muscles for ten to fifteen minutes twice daily. Put the ice in a plastic bag or use an ice bag from a medical supply store. Never apply the ice directly to your skin or you might experience more than osteoarthritis pain. Some of my patients get the best relief by alternating the icing sessions with moist heat. Whatever you choose, find the method that brings you the greatest reduction in pain and inflammation but is also convenient.

Step 2: Exercise Your Joints

"Exercise each day? I can hardly get out of bed." That is what my patients say to me when I stress the importance of exercise to end pain and gain mobility. Yet I also know that those who improve the most are the ones who exercise daily.

Why Exercise?

The purpose of exercise in arthritis is twofold. First, it will help improve the flexibility of your joints and keep them from becoming stiff and immovable. Second, exercise will help strengthen the muscles that support your joints. When your joints have strong muscles supporting them, they are less subject to inflammation, pain, and stiffness. Did you know that each year, between ages thirty and seventy, you could lose about 1 percent of your muscle strength? The loss is most noticeable at about age sixty. By age seventy, you may have lost up to 40 percent of your peak muscle strength. Weaker muscles mean your joints are not well supported. This combination can throw off your balance, giving you poor protection against falls and fractures.

What Exercise?

No matter what Super Aspirin or breakthrough medication you take or how much moist heat you use, the only way to make muscles stronger is through exercise. The best exercise is one that strengthens the muscles around joints without putting too much stress on the injured joint.

The type of exercise you choose will greatly depend on the type and location of your arthritis. For example, swimming is excellent for osteoarthritis in the hips and knees, because it strengthens the muscles around the joints while placing little stress on the joints themselves. Swimming also benefits those with rheumatoid arthritis, because water exercises help reduce all-over body pain. Other types of arthritis such as fibromyalgia benefit greatly from stretching exercises, which decrease the deep muscle pain and increase flexibility.

Some of the best forms of exercise include:

- Stretching and range-of-motion exercises

- Walking, biking, or other aerobic activities

- Weight lifting or resistance training

- Finger exercises, such as knitting or playing the piano

Common daily activities count as exercise, too, whether you are climbing stairs, raking leaves, walking at the mall, or sweeping your floors.

Stretching and Range-of-Motion Exercises

Stretching and exercises that move your joints in their full range of motion help you stay flexible and reduce pain. You can easily do the following exercises twice daily, working up to twenty repetitions each time. These are just a few examples of stretching and range-of-motion movements; ask your doctor or physical therapist for more range-of-motion exercises.

Start Slowly   It's okay to begin by doing just one to two repetitions of each range-of-motion exercise on the next pages. If you do these first thing in the morning after applying moist heat or taking a warm shower, and then at night after using moist heat again, you are well on your way to reducing pain. So many people think that if they cannot run a mile or two, their activity does not constitute "exercise." As one patient said, "I'd rather not exercise at all than lift my arms up and down twenty times." That patient still has incredible pain, too! Start slowly, gradually increase, and one day you may be walking that mile or two.

Once you can comfortably do several repetitions of each exercise, gradually increase until you reach twenty repetitions, twice daily. I have found this to be the optimum level that helps most arthritis patients maintain excellent strength and flexibility. This might take several months to achieve. Of course, if you feel pain during exercise, stop and talk to your doctor.

I suggest that you do stretching or range-of-motion exercises in the warm shower, bath, or whirlpool or immediately after moist heat to allow the most mobility with the least pain. And you may find it helpful to add moist heat *again* after exercise to decrease pain and stiffness in muscles and joints.

As you increase your level of exercise and fitness, it's important to not give up. Think of your commitment to a daily exercise program as one positive step you can take to end arthritis pain, one that takes time. The more you see your exercise time as equally important to your life as taking medications or even eating a healthful diet, it will become easier, more natural, and a part of your daily routine.

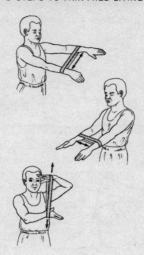

Figure 9.2

Shoulder Isometric Exercise Isometric exercises, such as the one in figure 9.2, use resistance to build muscle strength and flexibility without moving the joints. Start with low resistance at first and gradually increase it as you feel comfortable.

Get a special elastic or rubber band from your physician or physical therapist and place it just above your wrists. Pull your arms apart toward the side of your body. When the band feels tight, giving resistance, hold for six seconds. Then pull your right arm upward and your left arm downward, and hold for six seconds. Reverse this, pulling your left arm upward and your right arm downward, giving resistance, and hold for six seconds. If it is not painful, slowly increase the time you hold the band in these positions.

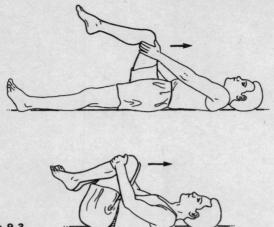

Figure 9.3

Hip Flexion Exercise These exercises stretch the hips, knees, and back. You can do these on the floor or on your bed.

Bend each knee to your chest, one at a time. If you need to, use your hands to help move your knee toward your chest. First bend your right knee to your chest, then your left. Repeat, alternating knees. Try to increase to five, then to ten, then up to twenty repetitions, twice daily.

Now pull both knees to your chest at the same time. Hold for six seconds and slowly rock from side to side while holding your knees to your chest, then gently bring your legs down. Repeat, gradually increasing to five, then ten, then twenty repetitions, twice daily.

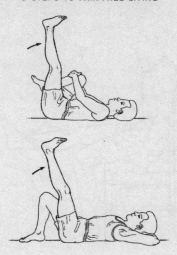

Figure 9.4

Straight Leg Raise This exercise strengthens the quadricep muscles at the front of the thigh; these muscles support the knee. The straight leg raise also strengthens your abdominal muscles and improves the flexibility of your legs. Lie on your bed or on the floor, whichever is more comfortable.

You can bend your knee slightly as shown, or hug one leg to your chest if you have chronic back pain from arthritis. Raise your other leg slowly while keeping your back flat on the floor or bed. Raise your leg as high as you can, but stop if your back begins to arch. Try to keep your abdomen tight. Hold and count to six. Lower your leg, then repeat the same for your opposite leg. Repeat for both legs, gradually increasing to five, then ten, then twenty repetitions, twice daily. If you have severe pain with this or any exercise, stop immediately and talk to your doctor.

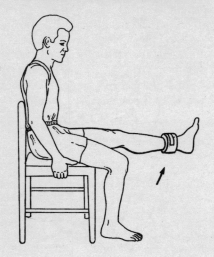

Figure 9.5

Weight Training

Many women still associate weight training with building bulky muscles, but this isn't the case. Weight training will help strengthen and preserve the muscle mass you already have and reduce your arthritis aches. Did you know that fat burns two to three calories per pound, while muscle burns fifty calories per pound?

A revealing Tufts University study found that people with rheumatoid arthritis could safely increase their strength by up to 60 percent with a modest weight-training program. Another study published in the *Journal of the American Medical Association* found improvements in arthritis when patients combined weight training with aerobic exercise. To gain the strengthening benefit without irritating the joints and causing further injury, proper technique is important. Check with your physician or consult a physical therapist to help design an exercise program that meets your specific arthritis needs.

Exercise Using Light Weights Try sitting in a chair with the weights strapped on your ankles. Straighten your knee, hold for a few seconds, and lower your foot to the floor. Repeat with the opposite knee, then gradually repeat up to five, then ten times, twice daily.

Start with 1 pound weights and gradually increase as you feel comfortable to 2 to 5 pounds on each ankle.

---

5 DAYS TO PAIN-FREE LIVING

....

Here's a five-day schedule for pain-free living to help you start using the moist heat and exercises twice a day—it must become a habit! After the first five days on the plan, repeat the routine, slowly increasing your exercise and activity as your pain lessens and mobility increases. Remember to take Super Aspirins or other medications at the times prescribed by your doctor.

DAY	TIME OF DAY	ACTION
Day 1	7:00 A.M.	Moist heat—10–15 minutes
	7:15 A.M.	Range-of-motion exercises (3 repetitions or more)
	8:00 P.M.	Moist heat—10–15 minutes
	8:15 P.M.	Repeat morning exercises, adding light stretching
Day 2	7:00 A.M.	Moist heat—10–15 minutes
	7:15 A.M.	Range-of-motion exercises (increase repetitions, if you can)
	7:30 A.M.	5–10-minute walk (treadmill or outside)
	8:00 P.M.	Moist heat—10–15 minutes

	8:15 P.M.	Repeat morning exercises, adding light stretching
Day 3	7:00 A.M.	Moist heat—10–15 minutes
	7:15 A.M.	Range-of-motion exercises (8 repetitions)
	7:30 A.M.	5–10 minutes on stationary bicycle
	8:00 P.M.	Moist heat—10–15 minutes
	8:15 P.M.	Repeat morning exercises, adding light stretching
Day 4	7:00 A.M.	Moist heat—15 minutes
	7:15 A.M.	Range-of-motion exercises (increase reps, if no pain)
	7:30 A.M.	10-minute walk (treadmill or outside)
	8:00 P.M.	Moist heat—15 minutes
	8:15 P.M.	Repeat morning exercises, adding light stretching
Day 5	7:00 A.M.	Moist heat—15 minutes
	7:15 A.M.	Range-of-motion exercises (15 repetitions)
	7:30 A.M.	10-minute swim or aquatic stretching exercise
	8:00 P.M.	Moist heat—15 minutes
	8:15 P.M.	Repeat morning exercises and light stretching

Step 3: Take the Right Medication

You may need to try a number of different medicines before you find the right one—that means the one that best relieves pain and stiffness with the least side effects. If you are using Super Aspirins, a traditional NSAID, or a prescribed pain medicine, try it at the correct dose for about two weeks. With any new medicine, it's a good idea to first try samples from your doctor or buy only a small (two-week) supply. If you haven't noticed any improvement by then, ask your doctor about trying a different one. As one of my patients said, ''Once I found the medicine that worked, I knew it within twenty-four hours. I felt so much better taking it, and this is the way I wanted to feel.''

Talk with your doctor about what medication works best for you. Then stay on this medicine as you continue to use moist heat and exercises. The combination of medication and those steps will help you gain the best relief.

What About Rheumatoid Arthritis?

Rheumatoid arthritis can damage and destroy your joints, and in some cases this destruction starts within the first few months. So if a medicine is not working, it's crucial that you let your doctor know so you can try a different treatment.

If you suffer from rheumatoid arthritis, you may consider changing to a Super Aspirin or traditional NSAID from your current medication. There are also slow-acting rheumatoid arthritis medicines, described in chapter 8, that take longer to work but may suppress your arthritis at an earlier stage than NSAIDs. These new rheumatoid arthritis medicines may take one to three months to show results, but they offer a 70 to 80 percent chance of improvement and increase the chance of complete control of your arthritis. You might compare this to turning off the gas on a stove rather than putting water on the fire.

Your doctor or arthritis specialist will help you choose which of the slow-acting medicines to try first. Try to be patient and see how the total treatment of moist heat, exercises, medication, and diet, along with complementary treatments, stops your arthritis pain. If there's still no improvement, consider one of the breakthrough medicines discussed in chapter 8.

Cortisone-Type Medications

For those with rheumatoid arthritis, I sometimes add a small dose of oral prednisone, which is a cortisone derivative and the strongest of the anti-inflammatory drugs. Prednisone helps to calm inflammation, so it can be extremely helpful when rheumatoid arthritis starts or when it flares up. Low doses of prednisone can be given safely for pain control until other treatments can take effect. Some other types of cortisone drugs used are listed below.

If 7.5 milligrams or more of prednisone is used for two months or longer, your doctor may want to take some precautions to prevent such serious side effects as osteoporosis. Other possible side effects of prednisone and other cortisone-type drugs if used at high doses or for a longer period of time are listed on page 117.

COMMONLY USED CORTISONE-TYPE MEDICATIONS

BRAND NAME	GENERIC
Deltasone, Meticorten, Orasone	prednisone
Medrol	methylprednisolone
Aristocort, Kenalog	triamcinolone
Decadron, Hexadrol	dexamethasone
Celestone	betamethasone

COMMON SIDE EFFECTS OF CORTISONE-TYPE MEDICATIONS

....

Weight gain

Fluid retention (edema)

Hypertension (high blood pressure)

Gastric irritation and bleeding

Peptic ulcer disease and other intestinal problems

Osteporosis (bone thinning)

Thin and more fragile skin, easy bruising

Acne

Delayed healing of cuts and wounds

Certain types of cataracts

Glaucoma

Increased chance of infection

Higher blood glucose (or aggravation of diabetes mellitus)

Suppression of normal cortisone production

Menstrual irregularities

Other muscle and bone problems

Depression and other mental health disorders

Increased body hair growth

Changes in blood triglycerides

Non-narcotic Medicines

Pain medications can be used for temporary relief of increased arthritis pain. I prefer the non-narcotic pain medicines, which are not habit forming and do not usually cause drowsiness. Some of the most common ones are listed on page 118.

COMMONLY USED NON-NARCOTIC PAIN MEDICATIONS (PRESCRIPTION)

....

BRAND NAME	GENERIC
Toradol	ketorolac
Ultram	tramadol

Narcotic Pain Relief

When your pain is more severe, you may need a stronger painkiller. If your doctor prescribes a narcotic, take it carefully according to the directions because it can be habit forming. Let your doctor guide you. Some of the most common narcotic pain medicines are listed below.

COMMONLY USED NARCOTIC PAIN MEDICATIONS (PRESCRIPTION)

....

BRAND NAME	GENERIC
Darvon	propoxyphene
Darvocet	propoxyphene with acetaminophen
Darvon Compound	propoxyphene with aspirin
Talacen	pentazocine with acetaminophen
Talwin	pentazocine
Tylenol #3, Phenaphen #3	codeine with acetaminophen
Tylox, Percocet, Roxicet	oxycodone with acetaminophen
Vicodin, Lortab, Lorcet	hydrocodone with acetaminophen

Muscle Relaxants

Muscle relaxants relieve pain from muscle spasms or muscle tightness and are commonly used for arthritis in the back or neck. Muscle relaxants should be taken only as needed, because some can be habit forming. All muscle relaxants can make you feel drowsy and make it difficult to concentrate.

COMMONLY USED MUSCLE RELAXANTS (PRESCRIPTION)

BRAND NAME	GENERIC
Flexeril	cyclobenzaprine
Parafon Forte	chlorzoxazone
Robaxin	methocarbamol
Soma	carisoprodol

Medicines for Chronic Pain

Some medicines help when pain is constant, especially in the back or neck. A group of medicines used in the past for depression often relieve pain when used in low doses. These doses are too low to help depression, but they do help pain. Side effects can include difficulty in urination, constipation, dry mouth, or dizziness. Some of those most commonly used are listed on page 120.

Antidepressant medications are useful also because chronic pain can lead to depression. If you have constant pain, feelings of sadness, or difficulty sleeping, talk with your doctor to determine if an antidepressant should be considered in your case.

COMMONLY USED ANTIDEPRESSANT MEDICATIONS FOR CHRONIC PAIN (PRESCRIPTION)

BRAND NAME	GENERIC
Elavil	amitriptyline
Norpramin	desipramine
Pamelor	nortriptyline
Paxil	paroxetine
Prozac	fluoxetine
Sinequan	doxepin
Tofranil	imipramine
Zoloft	sertraline

Local Injections

Your doctor may also use local cortisone injections in the swollen arthritic joint to improve your pain and avoid many of the side effects of cortisone. You will feel improvement within a few days that may last as long as four to eight weeks. Injections are especially beneficial when one or two joints are much more swollen and painful than other joints or if the moist heat, exercises, and NSAIDs do not give enough relief. There are usually no serious side effects from injections. The cortisone injection in the joint should have little effect on the rest of your body.

Step 4: Change Your Diet

Study after study reveals that what you eat—or don't eat— will determine how your body protects you from illness, despite the state of your present health. With arthritis or any chronic illness, eating a healthful diet with a variety of foods such as dairy, vegetables, fruits, soy products, lean meats, and whole grains can help boost your immunity. Maintaining a normal weight is also crucial to reducing pain and staying active with arthritis. Look through the suggestions in this step to see what dietary changes you need to make.

Maintain a Normal Weight

Being overweight increases your risk of osteoarthritis and puts unnecessary stress on inflamed joints. Some studies show that those who are overweight in their twenties have a greater risk of arthritis later in life. The good news is that patients who lose weight often notice less knee and hip pain and stiffness. Aim to lose a half-pound per week, and when you've lost ten pounds in five months, your arthritis pain may greatly improve. Gradually increase your walking, stationary biking, or swimming until you achieve your weight-loss goal. Talk with your doctor or certified nutritionist and see what type of dietary plan would work best for you.

Find Your Body Mass Index

How do you know what your goal weight should be? The body mass index (BMI), based on new guidelines issued by the National Institutes of Health, helps estimate the amount of body fat you have by using a formula based upon your actual weight and height.

Using figure 10.7, locate the height closest to your height in the left-hand column. Starting at that height, run your finger along the horizontal line until you find the weight closest to your weight. Go up the column to find your BMI. If your BMI is 30 or above, you are considered obese by these new standards. Those with a BMI of 25 to 29.9 are considered overweight. Under 25 is probably a safe weight for you, but check with your doctor to make sure. If your BMI is too high, work with a certified nutritionist and formulate a safe weight-loss plan, basing your daily meals on the selections in the Food Guide Pyramid (figure 10.6).

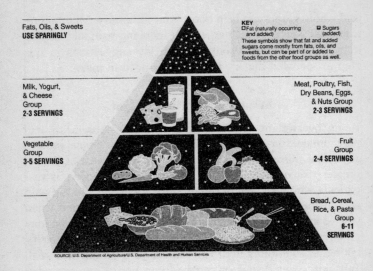

Figure 10.6 Food Guide Pyramid

Add Vitamins and Minerals

Nearly all nutrients play some role in helping your body reduce inflammation and pain, but antioxidants are crucial. These nutrients neutralize free radicals that can damage the body's cells and accelerate aging and cause diseases such as cancer. Some crucial ones are:

- Carotenoid (including beta-carotene): speeds up wound healing; found in many yellow, orange, or red fruits and vegetables, and in green leafy vegetables

- Vitamin C: helps to protect from infection; important in the production of collagen, the major support protein of cartilage

Figure 10.7 BODY MASS INDEX CHART

HEIGHT (INCHES)	19	20	21	22	23	24	25	26	27	28	29	30	31	32	33	34	35
58	91	96	100	105	110	115	119	124	129	134	138	143	148	153	158	162	167
59	94	99	104	109	114	119	124	128	133	138	143	148	153	158	163	168	173
60	97	102	107	112	118	123	128	133	138	143	148	153	158	163	168	174	179
61	100	106	111	116	122	127	132	137	143	148	153	158	164	169	174	180	185
62	104	109	115	120	126	131	136	142	147	153	158	164	169	175	180	186	191
63	107	113	118	124	130	135	141	146	152	158	163	169	175	180	186	191	197
64	110	116	122	128	134	140	145	151	157	163	169	174	180	186	192	197	204
65	114	120	126	132	138	144	150	156	162	168	174	180	186	192	198	204	210
66	118	124	130	136	142	148	155	161	167	173	179	186	192	198	204	210	216
67	121	127	134	140	146	153	159	166	172	178	185	191	198	204	211	217	223
68	125	131	138	144	151	158	164	171	177	184	190	197	203	209	216	223	230
69	128	135	142	149	155	162	169	176	182	189	196	203	209	216	223	230	236
70	132	139	146	153	160	167	174	181	188	195	202	209	216	222	229	236	243
71	136	143	150	157	165	172	179	186	193	200	208	215	222	229	236	243	250
72	140	147	154	162	169	177	184	191	199	206	213	221	228	235	242	250	258
73	144	151	159	166	174	182	189	197	204	212	219	227	235	242	250	257	265
74	148	155	163	171	179	186	194	202	210	218	225	233	241	249	256	264	272
75	152	160	168	176	184	192	200	208	216	224	232	240	248	256	264	272	279
76	156	164	172	180	189	197	205	213	221	230	238	246	254	263	271	279	287

BODY WEIGHT (POUNDS)

- Vitamin E: important for maintaining cell membranes; may exert beneficial effect in treating osteoarthritis and help to prevent damage to cartilage

YOUR ANTIOXIDANT HEALING TEAM

BETA-CAROTENE	VITAMIN C	VITAMIN E
apricots	broccoli	almonds
asparagus	cantaloupe	corn oil
beef liver	cauliflower	corn-oil margarine
broccoli	kale	cod-liver oil
cantaloupe	kiwi	hazelnuts
carrots	orange juice	lobster
kale	papaya	peanut butter
spinach	red, green, or yellow peppers	safflower oil
sweet potatoes	sweet potatoes	salmon
watermelon	strawberries	sunflower seeds
yellow corn	tomato juice	walnuts

Because some types of inflammatory arthritis are caused when the immune system goes haywire, it makes good sense to do all you can to keep your immune system functioning at its peak. The mineral zinc helps boost your immunity; calcium and magnesium can relax tense muscles. In addition, phytochemicals, nutrients found in foods called coumarins (found in limes, carrots, and oranges), keep your blood clotting and your immune system healthy. Lycopenes, found in the red pigment of tomatoes and red grapefruit, may also oost your body's immune function. Blood-thinning agents ccur naturally in garlic, onions, turmeric, and ginger.

Other vitamins and minerals needed for the synthesis of ormal collagen and maintenance of cartilage structures inlude vitamins A, B_5, B_6, zinc, boron, and copper. Patients ith rheumatoid arthritis may benefit from supplements of elenium, which reduces the production of inflammatory rostaglandins and leukotrienes. You can get adequate mounts of these and other important vitamins and minerals y taking a daily vitamin-mineral supplement. Ask your doctor to recommend one that will meet your individual needs.

The Antioxidant Power of Tea

oth green and black teas are also naturally rich sources of avonoids. Some recent studies indicate that the antioxidants a tea are more potent than those found in many fruits and egetables and may help prevent liver, pancreatic, breast, ıng, esophageal, and skin cancers. Tea can also help reduce ıe risk of cardiovascular disease and stroke, and some new ıudies indicate that it may help prevent osteoporosis. Scienısts have found that the intake of a single dose of tea inreases total antioxidant activity in the blood.

Up until now, most research has been done on green tea, lthough black tea is the most widely consumed worldwide. Iore results show that black tea, because it is derived from ıe same plant as green tea and thus has a similar chemical omposition, possesses comparable antioxidant activity to reen tea. So I encourage my patients to drink the tea that ıey enjoy.

More Healing Nutrients

ioflavonoids: Hosts of experiments have found that bioflaɔnoids increase immune system activation, which may proct you from inflammatory types of arthritis. Bioflavonoids ʳe in green peppers, lemons, limes, oranges, cherries, ʳapes, seeds, and nuts, and in the pulp and white core that ıns through the center of citrus fruits.

Quercetin: This highly concentrated form of bioflavonoid is found in citrus fruits, red and yellow onions, and broccoli. Some studies indicate it may benefit those with gout because it inhibits uric acid production in a similar way as the drug allopurinol. It also inhibits the release of prostaglandins, the inflammatory compounds.

Pycnogenol: Pycnogenol, a natural free-radical scavenger and antioxidant, reportedly helps reduce inflammation. Some studies show that pycnogenol is fifty times more potent than vitamin E and twenty times more potent than vitamin C.

Plant-based phytochemicals: Phytochemicals are biologically active substances that give plants their color, flavor, odor, and protection against plant disease. Phytochemicals work as potent antioxidants and are valuable to keep your immune system strong. Food sources of phytochemicals include apples, apricots, broccoli, Brussels sprouts, cabbage, carrots, cauliflower, garlic, legumes, onions, red peppers, soybeans, sweet potatoes, and tomatoes.

BENEFITS OF RED WINE

....

Some new studies suggest that trans-resveratrol, a natural compound found in red wine, may offer new hope for reducing the pain of arthritis sufferers. Researchers have found that trans-resveratrol blocks the activation of the COX-2 enzyme.

Trans-resveratrol is a substance produced in the skin of grapes to protect against oxidation and fungal infection caused by external stresses, such as temperature extremes and ultraviolet light. Trans-resveratrol is found in high concentrations in red wine, though its levels vary depending on the particular wine. Previous studies have identified trans-resveratrol as a powerful antioxidant, more potent than vitamin E, and suggest that it may also have anticancer and anti–heart disease properties.

This natural food substance is the first compound identified that both blocks the COX-2 enzyme and also inactivates the enzyme created by it. Some believe that trans-resveratrol may turn out to be an improvement over aspirin in fighting diseases associated with COX-2, such as arthritis.

Omega-3 Fatty Acids

New scientific studies have reported that eating fish such as salmon, mackerel, herring, and sardines, or taking fish oil capsules may help reduce inflammation that stems from arthritis. According to researchers, it's the omega-3 fatty acids that enable the body to make more products that help decrease inflammation. Studies have shown that when people affected by rheumatoid arthritis are given omega-3 fatty acids, found primarily in cold-water fish, pain and stiffness are reduced.

There are no specific guidelines on the exact dosage of fish oil, but experts believe that an effective daily dose may be three to five grams of the acids. You can also purchase capsules of eicosapentaenoic acid (EPA), which is available without a prescription at drug stores or health food stores. Or, if you'd rather get ample omega-3 fatty acids through your diet, you can eat fish several times a week. But this isn't an instant pain reliever; it takes twelve to sixteen weeks on omega-3 therapy before you feel benefits.

FISH HIGH IN OMEGA-3

....

anchovy	salmon
bluefish	sardines
capelin	shad
dogfish	sturgeon
herring	tuna
mackerel	whitefish

The Arthritis Diet

Some of my patients follow and find success with the so-called arthritis diet, which has been passed down through generations. This is an alkaline diet used for the treatment of osteoarthritis, rheumatoid arthritis, fibromyalgia, and other conditions where overacidity is thought to play a part. Naturopaths believe that arthritis is caused by the accumulation of toxic acids in the joints. These acids are thought to originate naturally in the intestine, but the body's metabolism fails to detoxify them when in excess in the diet.

I do suggest that if you try any food-restrictive diet, be sure to check with your physician or nutritionist about nutrition supplements that you may need. (I discuss the diet-arthritis link further on p 130.)

FOODS TO AVOID	FOODS TO EAT
Red meat	White fish, lentils, peas, chicken, eggs (no more than four per week)
Cow's milk, cheese, yogurt	Goat's milk, cheese, soy products
Brown, white wheat flour	Oats, brown rice, corn, buckwheat, millet, 100 percent rye-crisp bread
Citrus fruit	All other fruit, tomatoes only twice a week, all vegetables
Dry roasted nuts	All other nuts, especially hazelnuts, almonds, cashews, soybeans, and walnuts
Sugar—and foods containing sugar—syrup, honey	Sugarcane, molasses, dried fruit, sugar-free products
Coffee, decaf coffee, cocoa, caffeinated tea, alcohol	Grain coffees, herbal teas, unsweetened fruit juices, vegetable juices
Salt, pepper, vinegar	Vegetarian broth cubes
Butter and margarine	Olive oil
Chocolate	Carob

Diet Tips from the Arthritis Foundation

The Arthritis Foundation is a nonprofit organization whose mission is to support research, find the cure for and prevent arthritis, and improve the quality of life for those with this disease. There are local chapters of the Arthritis Foundation in most major cities. To help you make healthy choices, the

Arthritis Foundation recommends the following diet guidelines:

- Follow the Food Guide Pyramid (page 122) as you plan meals.

- Because protein is sometimes lost during the inflammatory process, if you have rheumatoid arthritis, eat 1 to 1.2 grams of protein per kilogram of body weight.

- If you take methotrexate for rheumatoid arthritis, add extra folic acid to help ease or prevent some of the side effects.

Food Additions

In a few studies, patients report feeling less pain and stiffness by adding the following foods to their diets. If you are not allergic to these foods, it would not hurt to try them.

- Cherries, blackberries, and blueberries, to help in cartilage formation and to prevent cartilage destruction.

- Garlic, onions, and cabbage, to increase the sulfur content of the body.

- Celery, parsley, apples, whole grains, alfalfa, ginger, and licorice, to balance immune function.

Step 5: Avoid Arthritis Triggers

New studies show identifiable triggers initiate arthritis in susceptible individuals, comparable to the way dust or pollen can trigger an allergy or asthma attack in certain people. So although it may be hard to pinpoint the exact causes of arthritis, if you know what might trigger arthritis flares or symptoms, you'll know what to avoid.

Identifying Food Triggers

I believe that the food-arthritis link has been too long ignored. Every day my patients tell me what foods they avoid to decrease pain—and how it really works for them.

Yet researchers have tested dietary triggers in a group of people with arthritis and found no conclusive evidence. In studies, red meat, fruit, dairy products, and preservatives were removed from people's diets for ten weeks. Although no major differences in scientific measurements were reported, two patients felt enough reduction in joint pain and stiffness to decide to continue the diet. I believe that to continue this strict deprivation diet, they must have felt much better!

Other studies have looked at wheat and other grains in the diet and added one type of food at a time to see its effect on arthritis. When wheat, milk products, or rice were added, some but not all persons noticed worsening of arthritis symptoms. There was no good way to predict which persons should avoid any single food item, but some definitely noticed a difference. These studies suggest that we may have individual sensitivities to certain food items.

Reading the Food Label

Reading food labels is important as you learn how foods may affect your arthritis pain and stiffness. Although government intervention has improved information provided to the consumer, it is important to know that there are still serious problems with food labels. For example, if the label reads ''egg substitutes,'' someone allergic to eggs may think this product is safe to eat. But although these substitutes may not contain the high-cholesterol yolk they may still contain egg whites, which can trigger a major allergic episode.

Products containing powdered sugar also contain cornstarch, a corn by-product that can trigger allergic reactions. Yet the food label may only say "powdered sugar," because ingredients present in very small amounts in foods are not required to be listed at all. For the person with osteoarthritis or rheumatoid arthritis who finds that such foods as peanuts, eggs, or corn products trigger pain and swelling, this misrepresentation on the label could result in an arthritis flare.

The Food Elimination Diet

So, how do you tell if a certain food triggers arthritis pain and stiffness? Although there are specific tests doctors can perform, mounting evidence has shown that an elimination diet is most valuable in identifying allergenic foods. This diet works by eliminating for two weeks the foods that most commonly trigger reactions. When symptoms subside, these foods are slowly reintroduced—one at a time—to see which ones trigger your symptoms.

Some common foods you will eliminate at first may include:

milk: butter, ice cream, yogurt, cheese, and other by-products

wheat: all breads, crackers, cookies, noodles, and other by-products

corn: grits, popcorn, corn chips, corn syrups, cornstarches, and by-products

citrus: oranges, grapefruits, lemons, limes, and other citrus fruits and juices

berries: strawberries, blueberries, raspberries

eggs

fish: including shellfish

peanuts: peanut butter or other products

tomatoes: pizza, spaghetti sauce, ketchup, and tomato by-products

yeast: dried fruits, vinegar, mushrooms, bread, pickles, beer

soybeans: soy sauce, soy lecithin, and tofu

- carob
- chocolate
- colas
- beans
- peas

Foods usually allowed during the elimination process include:

- **fresh poultry**
- **fresh meats**
- **vegetables** (except the listed varieties)
- **fruits** (except the listed varieties)
- **rice cereals**
- **water**

If you are instructed to reintroduce corn, you would eat only a small amount of corn at first, because a reaction could occur. If you have no reaction with the introduced food, you can eat it again in slightly larger amounts. You should also try by-products of the food to see if these are well tolerated. If there is no change in your symptoms and the food is tolerated, with your doctor's instruction you can go to the next category and reintroduce another food. If symptoms do develop, the new food should be stopped immediately.

If you have a suspicion that your arthritis flares when you eat certain foods, it may be worth your time and trouble to try at least a partial elimination diet. One patient stopped dairy products only and found her pain decreased after a period of three weeks. There is no other way to find out for sure, and if your arthritis improves, it will be worth it.

Food-elimination diets should be tried under the careful supervision of a physician or licensed nutritionist. You will need to ensure that the remaining foods in your diet during this period supply you with adequate nutrition.

COMMON FOOD ALLERGENS

....

alcohol (e.g., wine containing sulfites or other allergens)

berries (usually strawberries, blueberries, raspberries)

eggs

fish (usually shellfish)

grains (commonly wheat, gluten, corn, and rye)

milk proteins

peanuts

peppers

soy

yeast

Avoid Sulfites and Molds

Sulfites, which are used in foods and drugs as preservatives, can trigger arthritis symptoms in some people. Such sulfites as bisulfite, potassium, metabisulfite, sodium bisulfite, and sodium sulfite are frequently used in many bakery products, dehydrated potatoes, corn syrup, shellfish, salad dressings, pickles, wine and beer, and dried fruits. Surprisingly, sulfites are also found in some prescription and nonprescription drugs.

If molds trigger your arthritis pain, certain foods may exacerbate your problem. Watch out for fermented foods such as beer, cider, sauerkraut, vinegar, and wine, and foods made with yeast, such as breads, rolls, and many bakery products. Cheese, sour cream, buttermilk, and mushrooms can also aggravate a mold allergy.

Does Rain Increase Pain?

Weather has been discussed in arthritis since Hippocrates. Many patients—60 to 70 percent of patients with chronic pain, including arthritis pain—notice worsening when weather changes. It's been hard to pin down any particular type of weather, good or bad. Yet those who are affected notice it almost all the time, while many don't feel any effect at all. This may be why there is such a controversy about the question of weather and arthritis. One recent Canadian study found no relationship between joint pain and weather.

Nonetheless, most patients with arthritis notice the highest level of pain during weather changes, especially just before a cold front or other system moves in. Patients tell us that barometric pressure, humidity, and temperature changes can affect their pain and stiffness. Some people even move to another climate to avoid bad weather and although they may find relief initially, usually after several months their old pattern of arthritis pain and stiffness returns. Studies have not identified any particular place to live to prevent arthritis pain and stiffness.

What usually matters for those who are affected by weather is the amount of change in weather—not whether it's cold, hot, damp, or dry—but how often it changes. Our recommendation is that if you find a location that improves your arthritis pain overall, consider living there. But moving to a new city before you've tested it for a few months might disappoint you unless you really wanted to live there anyway!

The Challenge of a Chronic Illness

Using this basic five-step program of moist heat and exercises twice daily, the correct combination of medicines, diet changes, and weight control and avoiding arthritis triggers, you will certainly notice decreased pain and improved mobility. Many of my patients find even more improvement by adding a complementary treatment such as bodyworks and massage, biofeedback, acupuncture, body-mind therapies, herbal treatments, and natural supplements. They report that these alternative methods, when used with the 5-step treatment program, can alleviate symptoms of stress and also ease arthritis pain.

Please be patient and stick with this plan until you begin to see results, which could take as long as three to four weeks. First you'll notice some improvement in flexibility and strength, then your pain and stiffness will gradually decrease, and you'll find that moving around becomes less painful again. If this doesn't happen, talk with your doctor so you can decide which medicine to try next. Remember that most successful treatments are found after trying a few different combinations—not many people find success with the first medicine they try. Don't stop until you've found the medication that helps you control the pain so you can get around and do the things you really want to do.

CHAPTER 10

Complementary Treatments
to End Pain

While your doctor has prescribed Super Aspirins or other medications to ease your pain, and you are following my 5-step plan, non-drug or alternative interventions may allow you to take less medication, as well as exercise more personal control over your health. Scientific research has shown that specific mind-body approaches may help speed production of new immune cells and control the damaging stress hormone cortisol. For example, the relaxation response helps reduce physical stress and negative thoughts while increasing your inner ability to manage pain. Biofeedback alerts you to stress symptoms before they cause injury to the body, and listening to soothing music reduces pain by interrupting the cycle of pain and subsequent muscle tension. Each of these benefits has a positive effect on your arthritis.

Remember, continuing the 5 Steps to Pain-Free Living outlined in chapter 9, along with the Super Aspirins or other medicine, is vital for optimal pain relief and healing. Be sure to get your doctor's approval before complementing your medication plan with *any* unproven alternative therapy. And keep in mind that some of these complementary forms of pain relief may work for you while others may not.

Bodyworks

I am a great proponent of any type of bodyworks to ease pain. Bodyworks—the use of touch and physical contact to stimulate healing—can help increase circulation, give relief from musculoskeletal pain and tension, act as a mind-body stress releaser, and improve flexibility and mobility. After a massage or manipulation, you may experience:

- heightened alertness

- less anxiety

- an increase in the number of natural "killer cells" in the immune system

- lower levels of the stress hormone cortisol

- sounder sleep

Many of my arthritis patients find that a gentle massage gives them great relief when muscles are tense or joints are achy. Sometimes you can massage your own painful muscle or joint by applying gentle pressure at the point of pain, then gently kneading it to loosen it up. Especially after a warm shower, this self-massage seems to benefit my patients.

Chiropractic

Many of my patients complement their medical care with chiropractic. In this type of bodyworks, the practitioner focuses on spinal manipulation, or spinal adjustments, to treat pain. Chiropractors relieve pain by increasing the mobility between spinal vertebrae, which have become restricted, locked, or slightly out of alignment. They use hand manipulations with gentle pressure or stretching, multiple gentle movements of one area, or specific high-velocity thrusts.

If you try chiropractic, you might experience quick relief immediately after manipulation or it may take weeks to feel the benefit. Like other treatments, sometimes it may not work at all. Whether or not you find relief through manipulation, it is important to continue with the moist heat, exercises, and the prescribed Super Aspirins or other medicines, if needed. If you have no reduction in pain, talk to your medical doctor about other treatments that may help you.

Acupuncture

Although acupuncture was introduced in the United States in the late 1800s, it has become increasingly popular in the past two decades. This complementary therapy is a form of stimulation to end pain or relieve symptoms.

It is believed that acupuncture—inserting and twisting tiny-gauge needles at different points on your body—causes you to release endorphins, the body's natural calming hormones, which may add to the feeling of relaxation. Acupuncture may also trigger a hormone that fights inflammation, which could explain why those with chronic neck or back pain have found relief through this treatment. Some studies even suggest that acupuncture may trigger the release of certain neural hormones, including serotonin, that also contribute to feelings of calmness.

Acupuncture is approved by the National Institutes of Health (NIH) for nausea during pregnancy, nausea and vomiting associated with surgery or chemotherapy, and postoperative dental pain. Yet the World Health Organization of the United Nations also includes arthritis, frozen shoulder, lower back pain, sciatica, and tennis elbow as ailments that may benefit from acupuncture.

The average treatment takes about twenty minutes to one hour and is given either daily or two to three times a week. You may have to go through a series of at least eight to ten treatments before deciding if this is effective for you. If you choose to use acupuncture to reduce pain, talk with your medical doctor. I encourage my patients who try acupuncture to choose a licensed practitioner who uses only disposable needles.

Biofeedback

Some of my patients who suffer from chronic arthritis pain consider biofeedback an excellent treatment for relaxation and pain relief. Biofeedback uses electronics to measure body responses associated with stress, such as heart rate or muscle contractions. It is based on the idea that when you are given information about your body's internal processes, you can use this information to control those processes.

If you decide to try biofeedback, you will be connected to a machine that informs you and your therapist when you are physically relaxing your body. With sensors placed over specific muscle sites, the therapist will read the tension in your muscles, heart rate, breathing pattern, amount of sweat produced, or body temperature. Any one or all of these readings can let the trained biofeedback therapist know if you are learning to relax.

The ultimate goal of biofeedback is to use this skill outside the therapist's office when you are faced with arthritis pain. If mastered successfully, biofeedback can help you control your heart rate, blood pressure, breathing patterns, and muscle tension when you are *not* hooked up to the machine.

Hypnosis

Several patients of mine have had excellent results using hypnosis to control pain. They have told me that if induced correctly, this intense state of focused concentration will produce a feeling of calm and improve one's confidence in handling the challenges of coping with pain every day.

Hypnosis is not for everyone, so I always recommend that my patients find a qualified clinical psychologist or psychiatrist to learn this complementary technique of pain management.

Herbal Therapy

Although not all natural remedies are always safe, herbs may offer some relief. In a test of an herbal formula mixing turmeric, boswellin, and withania somnifera, researchers reported improvement in patients with rheumatoid arthritis. Study volunteers had less pain and swelling and improved mobility than those who took a placebo. Although this is only one trial, it may be the first of several combinations of herbal remedies proven to offer a positive benefit without negative side effects.

Before you take any of these herbs, talk with your doctor. Some herbs have sedative or blood-thinning qualities that may interact dangerously with NSAIDs or other arthritis medications. Others may cause gastrointestinal upset if taken in large doses. For example, ginkgo biloba may cause nausea, diarrhea, stomach upset, and vomiting if taken in larger doses and may reduce blood clotting time. Anyone taking Coumadin should not take this herb.

Ask your doctor about the following herbs, and if you decide to use herbal therapy, follow the package directions for appropriate dosage.

HEALING HERBS

HERB	PROPERTY
Astragalus	Stimulates immune function, stimulates production of interferon in fighting disease
Black current seed oil	Anti-inflammatory
Boswellia	Anti-inflammatory and improved blood supply to joint tissues
Devil's claw	Anti-inflammatory and pain relief

Echinacea	Anti-inflammatory, prevents infection, stimulates growth of new tissue
Feverfew	Prevents pain and swelling, anti-inflammatory
Garlic	Reduces fever, increases strength and energy
Ginger	Anti-inflammatory, increases stamina, blood thinner
Ginseng	Increases energy and immune response, decreases stress
Gotu-kola	Alleviates mental fatigue, reduces blood pressure, increases energy, nerve tonic
Kava	Reduces anxiety and calms nerves
Meadowsweet	Aspirinlike quality, anti-inflammatory
Mullein	Soothes inflammation, relieves pain
Passionflower	Mild tranquilizer, eases insomnia and stress, relieves pain
Pine bark	Stimulates circulation, reduces inflammation
St. John's wort	Calming, sedative, improves sleep, heals wounds, treats inflammation and pain
Wild lettuce	Mild sedative effect, relieves pain and insomnia

Natural Supplements

Natural dietary supplements include vitamins, minerals, herbs, and amino acids as well as natural enzymes, organ tissues, metabolites, extracts, or concentrates. Some of my patients have found great pain relief using supplements. My personal feeling is that if the supplement is safe and you are staying on your overall treatment plan, there's no harm in trying it. But be sure to ask your doctor if the supplement could affect the medications you may be taking. Most natural supplements are available at drugstores, grocery stores, or natural health food stores.

Glucosamine and Chondroitin

Glucosamine and chondroitin are two substances the human body produces to make cartilage. In supplement form, glucosamine comes from crab shells, and chondroitin comes from cow cartilage. Once glucosamine is taken, researchers have found that it goes to the cartilage in joints. In some studies, patients who took glucosamine had more than 50 percent decrease in their rating of pain, and in some cases, it was found to be the same or better in relief of symptoms than ibuprofen.

Glucosamine and chondroitin appear to have no side effects, although their long-term safety has never been established. Researchers do not know whether you must take the two supplements together or if one is effective taken by itself. It is all right to combine them because there are no known side effects of glucosamine when taken at doses recommended on the package. Please note, however, that there's no research on the safety of combining these supplements with Super Aspirins or with the other new arthritis medications.

If you have arthritis, this natural solution may provide some benefit. Nonetheless, keep in mind that you may have to stay on these supplements for several weeks to a month before you notice a decrease in pain and stiffness. I tell my patients that it's fine to try this alternative treatment, determine if there's any improvement over a few months, and continue it if you experience less pain and stiffness.

Stress Reduction

Living with any chronic illness causes stress, which can activate pain and anxiety. However, researchers also know that the brain makes its own morphinelike pain relievers, called endorphins and enkephalins. These hormones are associated with a happy, positive feeling and can help relay "stop pain" messages to the body's arthritic points. Studies show that when you can create a strong mental image using relaxation therapies, you actually feel "removed" from cumbersome stress and the pain response. This *mindfulness,* or focusing all attention on what you feel at the moment, can help you move beyond the pain you may feel as you become centered in a world of health and inner healing.

Resilience

We all have to live with some stress in our lives, but we can determine how we react to that stress. I suggest to my patients that they consider how someone with a resilient personality would handle a situation. Resilient people have fewer and less severe illnesses. Arthritis specialists know that patients with severe rheumatoid arthritis who have resilient personalities cope better than those who don't.

How can you make yourself more resilient? Suggestions from experts include:

- Maintain a sense of control. This means an ability to face future situations with determination rather than helplessness.

- Be a survivor. When problems happen, find ways to take action and prepare to survive the problem.

- Stay involved. Don't allow yourself to become withdrawn.

- Make a commitment to stick with healthy habits.

- Keep your activity at the highest level possible within your personal limits.

- Be determined. Don't let arthritis pain stop your activities.

- Look for areas of growth and opportunity. Though you may not be as active as in the past, there is a world of opportunity for you to use your talents and energy.

Psychotherapy

Coping with a chronic disease isn't easy—as you well know. Psychological intervention can be an excellent way to learn coping skills.

You might consider the following treatment options:

- *Individual counseling:* In a one-on-one session with a therapist, you can talk openly about problems you may have coping with your arthritis and use this time to vent frustrations or problems that need to be solved. The therapist may suggest ways to alleviate your depression, anxiety, or stress.

- *Family counseling:* Arthritis pain often extends beyond you and affects your family as well. Therefore, it is often helpful for family members to understand and accept your limitations and the possible impact this may have on your family's lifestyle. Family counseling may help you discuss the problems you have and get help accomplishing activities of daily living.

- *Group counseling:* There is no one who can better understand you than another person who "feels your pain." In group sessions led by trained therapists, you can share your feelings as well as develop effective coping strategies. The exchange of ideas at group sessions is often the most productive way to revamp your thought processes.

■ *Support groups:* In a support group, you can share
your feelings with others suffering from similar problems and comfort and encourage each other. The group
members can discuss the latest available treatments and
coping suggestions while affirming each other's positive experiences. The realization that "someone else
knows what I'm going through" is helpful as people
share their struggle living with arthritis. Call your local
chapter of the Arthritis Foundation for support groups
in your area.

Keep in mind that support groups are not meant to
be professional therapy groups. Those who would benefit from standard psychological or psychiatric intervention should seek professional treatment to fit their
needs.

Stress Reducers

Try the following alternative therapies to learn how to relax
on days when your pain seems to be more than you can
tolerate.

Relaxation Response

Set aside a period of about twenty minutes each day that you
can devote to relaxation practice, removing any outside distractions that can disrupt your concentration. Recline comfortably so that your whole body is supported. Use a pillow
or cushion under your head if this helps. Be sure to position
yourself so that you are relaxed without causing pain on any
arthritic joints.

During the twenty-minute period, remain still. Focus your
thoughts on the immediate moment and try to imagine that
every muscle in your body is becoming loose, relaxed, and
free of any excess tension. Concentrate on breathing in a
rhythmic fashion and making your breathing slow and even.
As you exhale each breath, picture your muscles becoming
even more relaxed, as if you breathe the tension away. At the

end of twenty minutes, take time to focus on your relaxed state. Notice whether muscles that felt tight and tense at first now feel loose and relaxed.

If practiced regularly, your body will learn to elicit the relaxation response and target the sympathetic nervous system. This in turn will help to relieve any anxiety that often accompanies postoperative pain. Many people find that it is only after several weeks of daily, consistent practice that they can maintain the relaxed feeling beyond the practice session itself.

Deep Abdominal Breathing

Mindful or deep abdominal breathing alters your psychological state, making a painful moment diminish in intensity. Think about how your respiration quickens when you are fearful or in great pain. Then consider how taking a deep, slow breath brings an immediate calming effect, reducing both stress and levels of pain. Although we take breathing for granted, it is one of the few bodily activities that we can consciously control. During deep abdominal breathing, you add oxygen to your blood and cause your body to release endorphins, while decreasing the release of stress hormones and slowing down your heart rate during painful times.

Lie on your back in a quiet room with no distractions. Place your hands on your abdomen, and take in a slow, deliberate, deep breath through your nose. If your hands are rising and your abdomen is expanding, then you are breathing correctly. If your hands do not rise, yet you see your chest rising, you are breathing incorrectly. Inhale to a count of five, pause for three seconds, then exhale to a count of five. Start with ten repetitions of this exercise, then increase to twenty-five, twice daily. Use this exercise anytime you feel anxious or stressed because of pain.

Progressive Muscle Relaxation

Progressive muscle relaxation involves contracting, then relaxing, all the different muscle groups in the body, beginning with your head and neck and progressing down to your arms, chest, back, stomach, pelvis, legs, and feet. To do this exercise, focus on each set of muscles, tense these muscles to the count of ten, then release to the count of ten. Go slowly as you progress throughout your body, taking as long as you can. Get in touch with each part and feel the tension you are experiencing. Also, notice how it feels to be tension free as you release the muscle.

Visualization

Visualization, or guided imagery, has been used successfully for controlling emotional distress, anxiety, and pain. To use this therapy, take a timeout in a quiet environment without distractions. Try to visualize a peaceful, relaxing scene, perhaps a vacation spot you have enjoyed in the mountains or at the seashore. Focus on this place, and try to recapture the moment as you imagine the sounds, smells, landscapes, and feelings you would experience. Become aware of your breathing and anxiety level as you focus, and do not let outside stimuli interrupt your imagery time.

Music Therapy

Some studies have shown that music can lower blood pressure and boost your immune cell count while reducing levels of stress hormones. If you listen to music for relaxation and pain reduction, avoid melodies that make you tense or that cause uneasiness. Spend ten to twenty minutes a day listening to soothing music, and try this in combination with another mind-body technique, such as guided imagery (visualization), deep abdominal breathing, or progressive muscle relaxation.

Aromatherapy

Some of my younger patients tell me they use aromatherapy to help ease the stress of a chronic illness. Studies on the inhalation of scents and stress relief, especially when combined with bodyworks or deep muscle massage, have been positive although not conclusive. One British study used aromatherapy on chronically ill patients and found that it did relieve stress, while other studies have shown that essential oils have an effect on brain waves and can also alter how you perceive stress.

Aromatherapy includes essential oils, extracts or essences that have been distilled or processed from a root, leaf, flower, seed, or even bark. Whether or not scents can reduce your arthritis pain depends on your response. In other words, if it works for you, use it! When inhaled, the aroma from essential oils stimulates a part of your brain that releases compounds said to help reduce stress, fight infection, and increase energy.

ESSENTIAL OILS FOR AROMATHERAPY

ESSENTIAL OIL	PROPERTY
Chamomile	Relieves insomnia, de-stresses, anti-inflammatory with massage
Lavender	Relieves insomnia, eases pain, de-stresses, anti-inflammatory, antibiotic
Orange	Increases energy
Peppermint	Increases energy, soothes nausea, antiseptic, anti-inflammatory
Rosemary	Increases energy
Vanilla	De-stresses

Ancient Mind-Body Exercises

Chi Gong (Qigong)

I am a strong proponent of chi gong, which I believe can help prevent and enhance the treatment of many chronic medical problems. After learning the series of exercises from an experienced practitioner, my wife, Linda, and I do these together each morning before work—in the comfort and privacy of our home. We have been practicing chi gong for almost one year.

Chi gong is based on the concept of balancing and complementing the life forces. It attempts to use the vital power "within" to help manage or control, among other things, medical problems, including arthritis. These exercises require different thinking than most of us have experienced in our Western culture, but it can be learned. For many people with arthritis, this can be a valuable alternative therapy to a basic treatment plan.

Tai Chi

The Arthritis Foundation reports that tai chi may be a perfect exercise for arthritis sufferers. In fact, this Chinese martial art appears to be safe for rheumatoid arthritis patients and may serve as an alternative for their exercise therapy and part of their 5-Step Treatment Plan. Some describe tai chi as "meditation in motion," with dramatic, flowing movements instead of forceful actions. If you need a full-body exercise yet find movement painful, tai chi may enable you to slowly move your body in a full range of motion, building strength and stability while also receiving the benefit of stretching and stress reduction. You can learn the movements in tai chi classes or from books and videos.

Yoga

The classical Indian practice of yoga is built on the foundation of ethics (yama) and personal discipline (niyama). It is used to relieve stress, achieve mind-body connectedness, and heal the body. Using deep breathing, concentration techniques, and body poses, you learn to calm your mind and increase flexibility and strength. Yoga postures can relieve mild aches and pains and decrease back pain.

To experience optimum results, yoga should be practiced

daily in the form of meditation and postures. You can learn yoga from a how-to book or instructional video, or join a yoga class at your local gym or YMCA.

What's Next?

What's next when medications and other treatment methods don't resolve your pain and stiffness? As I explain in the next chapter, you may want to consider surgery. After reading chapter 11, talk with your doctor to see if surgery is a viable pain-relieving alternative for you.

When Surgery
Is Necessary

Arthritis discomfort can be all too familiar, from osteoarthritis knee pain to the penetrating ache of tennis elbow or the fatigue of fibromyalgia. If your arthritis pain keeps you from enjoying an active lifestyle, I consider that a major, even life-threatening problem. What happens if you don't find enough relief from arthritis pain and inflammation using Super Aspirins or other medications, exercise, and moist heat applications? If your pain still persists, you might consider surgery as a viable treatment alternative.

Making the Decision

Surgery may be necessary if your pain is constant or severe, or if your joint has become very limited by arthritis despite treatment. For example, in osteoarthritis, the knee or hip cartilage may be so damaged that no medication will help. Or in rheumatoid arthritis, there may be so much swelling and thickening of the joint lining that medications may not be effective. The various surgeries used for arthritis, which I describe in this chapter, can help relieve the pain and let you be active again.

Are You a Good Candidate?

To decide if you are a good candidate for surgery, you must consider the level of pain you feel and how it has affected your quality of life. I always tell my patients that if their pain is constant and incapacitating and activity or exercise is limited *even with good medical treatment,* then surgery may be a consideration. A question I always ask patients to consider is: "What if you had *no* pain in the knee (or hip or shoulder)?" If your quality of life, including exercise and pain level, would be excellent with less pain, then surgery might be beneficial. But if you are able to do the things you want to do and keep your pain minimal, stay with the nonsurgical treatments.

Who Do You Call?

Surgery for osteoarthritis in the knee, hip, or shoulder or to remove a ruptured or herniated disc is now routinely done at most medical centers (a partial list is in the Resource Section on pages 174–76). Ask your arthritis specialist for names of excellent surgeons, as well as hospitals and outpatient surgical facilities. Check with your health care provider to see if the professionals and services needed will be covered under your insurance plan.

To keep the complications or risks of surgery low, check with your primary care physician or internist to make sure other considerations, such as heart problems, lung disease (chronic obstructive pulmonary disease or asthma), chronic illnesses like diabetes, or your age, do not put you at high risk for surgery. Let your doctor guide you as you make the safest choice.

What Type of Surgery?

Some important considerations when you decide about the type of surgery include:

- your age

- which joint is affected

- what you expect the new joint to be able to do (exercise and activity)

- how much cartilage loss there has been

- recuperation time in the hospital, rehabilitation center, or at home

- length of time for physical therapy or other exercises for recovery

Although the most common types of arthritis surgeries are total joint replacement and arthroscopy, there are now other choices available, depending on your individual needs. Some types of surgeries such as arthroscopy for osteoarthritis or rheumatoid arthritis are intended to give temporary relief or to avoid a bigger or more complicated operation. Yet often the results of these surgeries last for years. The total joint replacement is meant to be a permanent solution, but sometimes this is not so. When your doctor suggests total joint replacement, be sure you discuss this thoroughly with both your doctor and the surgeon to make sure it is the right choice at the right time.

It's important to keep in mind that surgery is actually the start of your new treatment regimen. After surgery, the difficult part will be making yourself follow your surgeon's prescribed exercise routine, including physical therapy and home exercises. You will probably be given one of the Super Aspirins or other new medications to halt pain and inflammation and to control arthritis in other joints.

The success of your exercise program often determines the overall success of the treatment. This is a great place to show your determination to improve your ability to be active and return to a better quality of life.

Osteoarthritis Surgery

Everyone's need for surgery to treat osteoarthritis pain is different. Let your physician and orthopedic surgeon guide you according to your particular joint and health concerns.

Arthroscopy

Especially if you need surgery for damaged cartilage in a joint, arthroscopy may be a viable option. It requires much less recovery time than other more involved types of surgery, and recovery from the surgery itself only takes a few days.

In arthroscopy, the surgeon will insert a thin fiber-optic scope into your joint to view it. In doing so, damaged cartilage and ligaments and other problems can be discovered. In many cases, the surgeon will be able to repair the abnormality at the same time, using the arthroscope. Physical therapy and exercises are critical to continue strengthening and improvement.

Arthroscopy and Debridement

For those with osteoarthritis in the joints, two procedures—arthroscopy and debridement—may help. Your surgeon will insert a thin, flexible fiber-optic scope into the joint through a tiny incision to remove loose pieces of cartilage, repair cartilage or ligament damage, or smooth the cartilage surface. Your surgeon can scrape the cartilage surface to try to stimulate new cartilage formation as the body heals the area. Physical therapy and exercises are important to complete your recovery with maximum improvement.

Osteotomy

This type of arthritis surgery is usually done on the knee, where the surgeon removes a small wedge of bone to correct a deformity. The procedure straightens the bones and returns the weight-bearing alignment to normal. Osteotomy allows for unrestricted physical activity once recovery has taken place, and I recommend it for patients younger than 50 years old to allow full activity while still leaving the choice of total knee replacement, if needed, for the future. In fact, 85 to 90 percent of my patients who have osteotomy experience good pain relief, which may last five to ten years.

Total Joint Replacement

You may want to consider this type of arthritis surgery if your arthritis pain is continuous and keeps you from being active. Ninety-five percent of patients who undergo joint replacement surgery respond with good pain relief in the replaced joint. In addition, joint replacement may increase your activity and improve your overall function in other joints.

Before you undergo total joint replacement, it's important to ask your doctor specific questions about your future activity level. Let your surgeon know the level of physical activity you want to enjoy, both in your leisure time and work. If you want to play tennis, golf, or garden, or you need to bend and lift for work, make sure your surgeon knows this ahead of time. You will be more satisfied with the results years after the surgery if both you and your physician understand your needs.

Total hip, shoulder, and knee joint replacements are routinely performed at most major medical centers.

Total Hip Replacement

There is no need for anyone to suffer from ongoing, severe pain or loss of use of the hip from osteoarthritis. Today's hip replacements have become so effective that in 95 percent of cases, patients can expect excellent pain relief. Your doctor will refer you to an orthopedic surgeon who can assess your hip damage and determine if you are a good candidate for total hip replacement.

New medical technology has greatly improved total hip replacement. One surgical method allows the bone to "grow" into the actual replacement part, without using cement. With this new technique, there's less of a chance of the once-common problem of loosening in the joint. Studies show that a repeat operation is needed in less than 2 percent of the surgeries using this method.

In some cases, bone loss around the artificial or replacement parts, which may occur after fifteen or more years, may necessitate a repeat operation or new artificial joint.

Total Knee Replacement

More than 50 million Americans suffer from knee problems that may result in wear and tear on the knee joint and osteoarthritis. Osteoarthritis in the knee can be extremely painful; for some sufferers, their pain level increases with each step. If you have unending pain and limited mobility even after following the basic treatment plan and taking Super Aspirins, you may want to talk to an orthopedic surgeon about total knee replacement. This cost-effective and successful way to treat osteoarthritis of the knee results in pain relief about 85 to 95 percent of the time.

Because osteoarthritis may affect one or two joints—but not all joints—the relief you feel from total knee replacement may improve your overall activity levels. If you had no knee pain, could you be more active and enjoy your life more? If you answered yes, and your treatment plan and Super Aspirins are not giving enough relief, then consider discussing this option with an orthopedic surgeon. This is also a viable option if you have a deformity of the knee along with severe and constant pain.

Depending on the health of the patient, total knee replacement can be performed in older patients, including those over age 70. If you are overweight, the doctor may suggest that you lose weight before the surgery to improve the chances for success.

Total Shoulder Replacement

While total hip and knee replacements are common operations for arthritis, joint replacement is used less frequently for the shoulder. Nonetheless, using the breakthrough surgical techniques developed in the past few years, your orthopedic surgeon can find the right treatment for you. In one recent study, more than 90 percent of osteoarthritis patients found satisfactory relief with improved range of motion, making activities such as washing their backs, reaching for a shelf, and combing hair much easier.

Hand Surgery for Osteoarthritis

When the basic treatment plan and Super Aspirins do not completely relieve the constant pain and loss of the use of your hand, several types of surgery are available. The surgeon may stabilize your joints with ligament and tendon surgery or perform surgery that fuses the joint, which helps control the pain yet may limit its movement. In some cases, when use of the hand is not as great, such as with older patients, the surgeon will use artificial metal and silicone implants.

Cartilage Transplants and Grafts

So far, no treatment has completely replaced or regrown normal joint cartilage. Growth factors that can encourage new cartilage growth after replacing normal cartilage cells may be just a few years away from discovery. However, several new procedures offer benefits today.

A cartilage transplant is a procedure for patients who have areas of joint cartilage damage from injuries, but not severe overall cartilage loss, such as with advanced osteoarthritis. The surgeon takes healthy cartilage cells from the patient's knees, grows them further in a lab, then replaces them back in the knee at the site of the damaged cartilage. If growth is successful, this may help repair joint cartilage and may help prevent osteoarthritis.

In some research, grafts of small pieces of cartilage have been moved from one area of the knee to another area where there was no cartilage. Successful cartilage grafts help replace the lost cartilage. The resulting pain relief may help delay another surgery, such as total joint replacement.

Other studies have found that grafts of a very thin portion of the outer layer of bone onto an area of damaged cartilage may help patients who have cartilage damage in the knees. There is evidence of some cartilage growth in these cases, and some patients even experience decreased pain and improved activity levels. This is done well before there is severe osteoarthritis with loss of cartilage throughout the joint.

Surgery for Rheumatoid Arthritis

Synovectomy

Surgery for rheumatoid arthritis may help restore good use of a joint or control pain. Fortunately, with the breakthrough medicines outlined in chapters 7 and 8, along with a regular treatment program, most patients can control their rheumatoid arthritis without surgery but if that's not the case for you your orthopedist can help you make the best decision regarding surgery.

In rheumatoid arthritis, the knees may not respond to medical treatment. Before there is severe cartilage destruction and loss, removal of the joint lining, called synovectomy, can give relief, sometimes for up to five years. Synovectomy is usually now done by arthroscopy. A fiber-optic camera is used to visualize the joint. At the same time the swollen joint lining is removed, cartilage damage may be repaired to improve knee movement. Because this is usually done as an outpatient procedure, recovery is quick, and physical therapy and home exercises can begin soon after surgery.

Synovectomy can also be used with rheumatoid arthritis in

the hands and wrists, when severe pain and swelling in the wrists or fingers do not respond to other medical treatment for at least six to nine months. It is used when there has been no joint destruction. The surgery can help the pain, increase use of the fingers or wrists, and usually improve the hand's appearance.

Total Joint Replacement

Just as in osteoarthritis, total joint replacement in rheumatoid arthritis can be effective for pain relief and improvement in use of the joint. Total joint replacement of the hip, the knee, and the shoulder are considered when cartilage and bone are destroyed by the rheumatoid disease and pain and stiffness are not controlled with medication and exercises. The procedures, same as those described on pages 156–158, provide good pain relief in more than 90 percent of cases.

Replacement of finger joints in rheumatoid arthritis can successfully control pain and improve the use of the hand. It can also correct the deformity caused by arthritis, though appearance is not the main objective—how your hand works and feels are what matters.

Other joint surgery is also available to treat pain and help return the use of your elbow, ankle, and foot. Discuss the specific choices for surgery with your orthopedic surgeon. Some joints may benefit from fusion (arthrodesis), which renders the joint immovable. This older type of surgery usually gives excellent pain relief and benefits joints such as the ankle. Patients who have ankle fusion performed are usually happy with the relief from arthritis pain.

Surgery for Back Pain From Osteoarthritis and Disc Disease

Lumbar Laminectomy/Discectomy

This open surgical procedure is done in two steps beginning with the laminectomy–open surgery that involves opening the spinal canal with an incision to see the pinched nerve root. The lamina, or bony arch of the vertebra, is removed, then the second procedure, discectomy, removes the herniated or bulging disc. Physical therapy and rehabilitation are almost as important as the surgery for full recovery and pain reduction.

Percutaneous Discectomy

With percutaneous discectomy, you will have even less trauma, pain, and bleeding and may even be able to walk out of outpatient surgery the very same day. Using local anesthesia and x-rays for guidance, your surgeon will begin with a small incision that allows placement of an instrument into the disc space to remove the disc. Unlike open surgery, which involves a large incision, muscle dissection, and bone removal, percutaneous discectomy requires only a puncture wound, where part of the ruptured disc is removed with suction. The downside is that the success rate of percutaneous discectomy can be lower than open surgery.

KTP Laser

Although not widely used, the KTP laser is another new technique. You might be a candidate for this if tests results show that you have a bulging but not yet herniated disc. The surgeon will place a needle into the disc, using a silicon optical fiber attached to a laser, which transmits energy into the disc and softens it. As the pressure inside the disc decreases, it will shrink and pull the bulge off the nerve root, helping to decrease pain.

Chemonucleolysis

Depending on the exact site of the disc, in the past surgeons injected a chemical (chymopapain) to dissolve the soft part of the ruptured disc. In some cases, this will help lessen the pressure on the nerve, although there are frequent allergic reactions to the drug. This method gives good pain relief in 60 to 80 percent of cases, but it is less popular because of reaction to the medication, and surgery is often required after this procedure.

Anterior Discectomy and Fusion for Cervical Disc Disease

This common method of disc repair is open surgery and calls for a large incision at the front of the neck, removal of the ruptured disc, then fusion or replacement with a bone graft, often from the pelvic area. This bone graft fuses the two vertebrae together and protects the spinal cord. But with this fusion, the stress is now distributed to all the other discs as the spine stiffens. This type of surgery may require you to wear a brace for a period of time during recovery and rehabilitation.

Interviewing a Surgeon

Medicine is changing dramatically. In years past we relied on our doctors to provide medical care and keep us well. However, the traditional, autocratic role of doctors is now challenged by millions of people as they seek to make informed choices regarding their bodies and necessary health care. Although you may feel uncomfortable interviewing a surgeon and asking pertinent, even personal, questions regarding his knowledge and experience, it is important to do this to find that professional whom you can trust.

Your primary care doctor or internist will recommend either a neurosurgeon or orthopedic surgeon. A neurosurgeon specializes in surgery on the nervous system, including the brain and spinal cord; an orthopedic surgeon focuses on bone and joint surgery. Both do surgery for certain arthritis complications. Once you have been given a referral, in this age of managed care you must check to see if this surgeon will be accepted by your insurance provider.

Over the telephone, you can find out if the surgeon is board certified, which means that the doctor passed a standard exam given by the governing board in her specialty, and where the doctor went to medical school. Your local medical society will provide this information. (Although this should not always be a determining factor, if you've never heard of the school you might do more research.) Sometimes it's a plus if the doctor is involved in academic pursuits such as teaching, writing, or research, because this surgeon may be more up to date in the latest developments in his field. It is important to know where the doctor has hospital privileges and where these hospitals are located. Some doctors may not admit patients to certain hospitals, and this is an important consideration, especially if you have a chronic health problem. You should consider how many surgeries this physician has done on arthritis patients with your specific problem. For example, to repair a herniated disc, twenty-five to thirty would be advisable.

During the examination, find out about the preferred method of surgery. Is he or she current in using the latest methods for surgery? Will patient-controlled analgesia (PCA) be considered? This means you control the amount of pain medication given after surgery. Ask if the surgeon will do all of the surgery. If not, how much will be done by the surgeon's assistant, physician's assistant, or hospital resident? Also, find out if this doctor will be on call after surgery, or if another doctor will see you.

And let's not forget to mention that with the increased demands on our health care system, anyone can make a mistake. There is only one way to reduce chances that this will happen to you: *be assertive and knowledgeable as you take responsibility for your health.*

Choose an Accredited Hospital

Depending on the type of surgery, the procedure may be done in your surgeon's office, or at an *outpatient* facility, where you are admitted for surgery, then leave the same day. Or, you may be admitted to a hospital for *inpatient* surgery. Usually the site will be your surgeon's recommendation, or the place where he or she has hospital privileges. Nonetheless, if your surgery is elective and if you have time, go to this outpatient facility or hospital, or ask around about its reputation.

Meet the Anesthesiologist

If your surgery is immediate, you may not have the chance to talk at length with your anesthesiologist. This professional maintains your life while the normal triggers for breathing are anesthetized. However, if you are planning ahead for surgery, it is standard to meet with this person during the preoperative exam. Whether you meet your anesthesiologist a week ahead or five minutes before surgery, make sure she knows the following:

- Whether you have rheumatoid arthritis or osteoarthritis

- Whether special precautions are needed because of rheumatoid arthritis affecting the neck

- Other health problems you may have (lung disease, heart problems, chronic illness)

- Problems with anesthesia in the past

- Your desire to be awake during surgery

Preparing for Surgery

If your final option for pain relief is surgery, it's important to know that each type of surgery has a specific advantage, depending on the severity and location of the problem and such factors as your age or other chronic illnesses.

- **Open surgery** generally requires a few days to a week in the hospital, general anesthesia, and three weeks to three months of recovery, including physical therapy.

- **Arthroscopy** requires much less recovery time than other more involved types of surgery.

- **Outpatient procedures** may allow you to leave the hospital within hours of surgery.

However, no matter how "minor" the procedure appears, you will still be expected to follow the doctor's orders on rehabilitation and physical therapy. You may still need to take one of the Super Aspirins or other new medications to keep inflammation down and halt pain. Be sure to let your doctor guide you as you choose the type of surgery that is best to help you end pain and regain an active life.

Conclusion

....

Living Pain Free

Using the information in this book, I hope you have learned more about the type of arthritis you have and how it might best be treated. Remember, the new Super Aspirins and other breakthrough medications are not meant to be temporary "cures" for arthritis pain. Rather, when combined with the ongoing basic treatment plan of moist heat, exercise, a nutritious diet, and avoidance of arthritis triggers, these medications can stop arthritis pain now and for years to come.

I like to tell patients that sticking with the Super Aspirins or other medication and your basic treatment plan is a process, not an end in itself. Changing behaviors over time, such as taking time daily to stretch, walking before work, or lingering in the warm shower for ten to fifteen minutes in the morning and at night to reduce pain, takes continuous commitment. (You must exercise and use moist heat twice a day—on both good days and bad.) Finding a complementary treatment that works well for you may also boost pain control.

I'd like to share some success stories excerpted from letters my patients have sent me about these miraculous medications and how they have helped change the way they feel.

Dear Dr. McIlwain:

    The new medication you gave me in the trial has changed my life! Before taking Celebrex, I could hardly go to church with my wife. Today, I am back gardening and even doing some fishing with my grandson. I cannot wait to wake up each day because I know I can really enjoy my life to the fullest.

Carl, 68

Dear Dr. McIlwain:

When the nurse suggested that I participate in the Vioxx trial for my osteoarthritis in the back and hips, I honestly wanted to say, "Why bother?" After living with this for years, nothing has ever helped before. But I did, and it worked. I was shocked. I kept thinking the pain was going to reappear or that my stomach would start aching as it did with the other NSAIDs—but none of this happened. Instead, I feel as if I stepped back in time twenty years.

Alice, 51

Dear Dr. McIlwain:

The new medicine, Arava, you gave me for my rheumatoid arthritis, has made me smile again. My family also thanks you! I wish every person with rheumatoid arthritis could feel as good as I feel.

Kenneth, 38

Dear Dr. McIlwain:

Who would have thought that a tiny tablet taken twice a day could change the way I feel so dramatically? The Super Aspirin is a miracle!!! I have no pain in my knees—and my stomach is not churning and bubbling like it did with other medicines. I'm even walking two miles a day on my treadmill—I knew you'd like to hear that!

Rita, 59

Dear Dr. McIlwain:

Remember the day you diagnosed me with rheumatoid arthritis? I will never forget how I went home and cried myself to sleep. I thought my world was over.

How would I care for my new baby and my husband? Then you called and told me about Enbrel. It was like a miracle. It wasn't long before I was back to my old self again, pushing Rebecca's stroller around the block and going out to eat with my family.

Enbrel virtually changed my life from being an invalid to being a young vital mother and wife again. Thank you so much!!

Karen, 34

Share Your Personal Story

I'd like to hear from you. Have you used one of the Super Aspirins or other breakthrough medications? Did you find relief from pain? Perhaps you are now controlling a weight problem or are able to be as active as you were a decade ago. Did any of the complementary treatments help you ease pain and increase mobility? Do you have a success story to share? If so, tell me all about it!

Write to me at:
OAStudy@aol.com
or
TMGstudy@aol.com

Appendix

....

Resources and Support Groups

American Society of Pain Management Nurses
7794 Grow Drive
Pensacola, FL 32514
(888) 34-ASPMN
(850) 484-8762 (fax)

American Academy of Orofacial Pain
19 Mantua Road
Mount Royal, NJ 08061
(609) 423-3629
(609) 423-3420 (fax)

American College of Rheumatology
1800 Century Place
Suite 250
Atlanta, GA 30345
(404) 633-3777
(404) 633-1870 (fax)
Website: http://www.rheumatology.org

American Society for Action on Pain
P.O. Box 3046
Williamsburg, VA 23187
(757) 229-1840
Website: http://www.druglibrary.org/schaffer/asap

American Pain Society
4700 West Lake Avenue
Glenview, IL 60025-1485
(847) 375-4715

(847) 375-4777 (fax)
Website: http://www.ampainsoc.org

American College of Osteopathic Pain Management &
Sclerotherapy
107 Maple Avenue
Silverside Heights
Wilmington, DE 19809
(302) 792-9280
(302) 792-9283 (fax)

American Chronic Pain Association
P.O. Box 850
Rocklin, CA 95677-0850
(916) 632-0922
(916) 632-3208 (fax)
Website: http://www.theacpa.org

American Society of Regional Anesthesia
P.O. Box 11086
Richmond, VA 23230-1086
(804) 282-0010
(804) 282-0090 (fax)
Website: http://server.tacticalsolutions.com

American Academy of Pain Medicine
4700 West Lake Avenue
Glenview, IL 60025-1485
(847) 375-4731
(847) 375-4777 (fax)
Website: http://www.painmed.org

American Academy of Pain Management
13947 Mono Way #A
Sonora, CA 95370
(209) 533-9744
(209) 533-9750 (fax)
Website: http://aapainmanage.org

Arthritis Foundation
1330 West Peachtree Street
Atlanta, GA 30309

(404) 872-7100
Website: http://www.arthritis.org

Centers for Disease Control 24-hour voice
information system on Lyme Disease
(888) 232-3228

FMS Support Groups
Fibromyalgia Alliance of America
P.O. Box 21990
Columbus, OH 43221-0990
(614) 457-4222
(614) 457-2729 (fax)

International Association for the Study of Pain
909 NE 43rd Street, Suite 306
Seattle, WA 98105-6020
(206) 547-6409
(206) 547-1703 (fax)
Website: http://www.halycon.com/isap

Lupus Foundation of America, Inc.
1300 Piccard Drive, Suite 200
Rockville, MD 20850-4303
(301) 670-9292
(800) 558-0121
Website: http://internet-plaza.net/lupus

National Institute of Arthritis and Musculoskeletal
and Skin Diseases
National Institutes of Health
Building 31, Room 4C32
31 Center Drive, MSC 2350
Bethesda, MD 20892-2350
(301) 496-8188
(301) 480-2814 (fax)
Website: http://www.nih.gov/niams

National Institute on Aging
NIA Information Center
P.O. Box 8057
Gaithersburg, MD 20898-8057

(800) 222-2225
Website: http://www.nih.gov/nia

National Chronic Pain Outreach Association
7979 Old Georgetown Road, Suite 100
Bethesda, MD 20814-2429
(301) 652-4948
(301) 907-0745 (fax)

The Neuropathy Association
60 East 42nd Street, Suite 942
New York, NY 10165
(212) 692-0662
Website: http://www.neuropathy.org

New England Pain Association
P.O. Box 11086
Richmond, VA 23230-1086
(804) 282-4011
(804) 282-0090 (fax)

Osteoporosis and Related Bone Diseases National
Resource Center
1150 17th Street NW, Suite 500
Washington, DC 20036
(202) 223-0344
(800) 624-BONE
TTY: (202) 466-4315
Website: http://www.osteo.org

Scleroderma Foundation
89 Newbury Street, Suite 201
Danvers, MA 01923
(978) 750-4499
(978) 750-9902 (fax)
(800) 722-HOPE (Help Line)
Website: http://www.scleroderma.org

The Scleroderma Federation
Peabody Office Building
One Newbury Street
Peabody, MA 01960

(508) 535-6600
(800) 422-1113
(508) 535-6696 (fax)

Trigeminal Neuralgia Association
P.O. Box 340
Barnegat Light, NJ 08006
(609) 361-1014
(609) 361-0982 (fax)
Website: http://neurosurgery.mgh.harvard.edu/tna

The Sjögren's Syndrome Foundation
333 North Broadway
Jericho, NY 11753
(800) 4-Sjogrens
Website: http://www.sjogrens.com

Spondylitis Association of America
(800) 777-8189
Website: http://www.spondylitis.org

The United Scleroderma Foundation, Inc.
P.O. Box 399
Watsonville, CA 95077-0399
(800) 722-HOPE

Internet Sites

http://www.aapainmanage.org
American Academy of Pain Management

http://www.aapmr.org
The American Academy of Physical Medicine & Rehabilitation

http://www.aaos.org/wordhtml/pat_educ.htm
American Academy of Orthopaedic Surgeons

http://www.rheumatology.org
American College of Rheumatology

http://www.ama-assn.org
American Medical Association

http://www.usdoj.gov/crt/ada/adahom1.htm
Americans with Disabilities Act

http://members.aol.com/bosaud/arthritis/arthritis.htm
Arthritis Internet Resource Center

http://www.pslgroup.com/arthritis.htm
Doctor's Guide to Arthritis Information and Resources

http://www.healthfinder.org
Healthfinder™

http://mediconsult.com
Mediconsult.com: The Virtual Medical Center

http://www.nof.org
National Osteoporosis Foundation (NOF)

http://www.aota.org
American Occupational Therapy Association, Inc.

http://www.medlib.iupui.edu/hw/rheuma/home.html
Rheumatology Page of HealthWeb

Teaching Hospitals

Here is a partial list of teaching hospitals.

Mayo Clinic Rochester
200 First Street, SW
Rochester, MN 55905
(507) 284-2511

Johns Hopkins Hospital
600 North Wolfe Street
Baltimore, MD 21287
(410) 955-5000

Hospital for Special Surgery
535 East 70th Street
New York, NY 10021
(212) 606-1000

Brigham and Women's Hospital
75 Francis Street

Boston, MA 02115
(800) BWH-9999
(617) 732-5500

The Kirklin Clinic
2000 Sixth Avenue South
Birmingham, AL 35233
(205) 801-8000
UAB HealthFinder at (205) 934-9999

UCLA Medical Center
10833 LeConte Avenue
Los Angeles, CA 90095
(800) 825-2631

Massachusetts General Hospital
55 Fruit Street
Boston, MA 02114
(617) 726-2000

The Cleveland Clinic Foundation
9500 Euclid Avenue
Cleveland, OH 44195
(216) 444-2200
(800) 223-2273

Duke Consultation and Referral Center
3100 Tower Boulevard
Suite 1300, Box 55
Durham, NC 27707
(919) 416-3853
(919) 403-4258

UCSF Stanford Health Care
300 Pasteur Drive
Stanford, CA 94305
(650) 723-4000

Barnes-Jewish Hospital
216 South Kings Highway Boulevard
St. Louis, MO 63110
(314) 747-3000
(314) 362-8877 (fax)

Parkland Health & Hospital System
5201 Harry Hines Boulevard
Dallas, TX 75235
(214) 590-8000

UVA Health Sciences Center
Charlottesville, VA 22908
(800) 251-3627

Northwestern Memorial Hospital
250 East Superior Street
Chicago, IL 60611-2950
(312) 908-8400

Assistive Devices for Arthritis

To learn more about occupational therapy, physical therapy, and assistive devices, contact the following:

Arthritis Devices

Accent on Living: Buyer's Guide
Accent on Living
P.O. Box 700
Bloomington, IL 61702
(309) 378-2961
Updated annually, this guide lists a multitude of items that are available for daily living tasks. Stores and resources are listed with contacts. It is a great resource for items that are hard to find.

Yes I Can
(888) 366-4226
E-mail: info@YesICan.com
This store's catalog is too large to mail. Salespeople will discuss assistive devices you are looking for and will mail or fax copies of pages from the catalog to you.

Arthritis Aids Catalogs

Maddak, Inc. Catalog
Maddak, Inc.
6 Industrial Road
Pequannock, NJ 07440-1993
(800) 443-4926
This free catalog offers equipment for daily living such as accessories for wheelchairs, eating utensils, and dressing aids.

ADL and Rehabilitation Product Guide
Fred Sammons, Inc.
P.O. Box 5071
Bowling Brook, IL 60440
(800) 323-5547
(800) 547-4333 (fax)
This free catalog offers equipment for daily living such as accessories for wheelchairs, walkers, eating utensils, and dressing aids.

AdaptAbility: Products for Independent Living
AdaptAbility
P.O. Box 515
Colchester, CT 06415-0515
(800) 243-9232
Ask for the AdaptAbility free catalog, updated annually, which lists items such as kitchen aids, household items, and bathroom support equipment—safety bars, transfer benches, stools, and more.

North Coast Medical AfterTherapy Catalog
Access to Recreation, Inc.
18305 Sutter Boulevard
Morgan Hill, CA 95037-2845
(800) 821-9319
(877) 213-9300 (fax)
This free catalog carries a wide assortment of daily living items, including wheelchair accessories, walkers, transfer boards, exercise equipment, eating utensils, and more.

Can-Do Products For Your Active Independent Life
Independent Living Aids, Inc.
27 East Mall
Plainview, NY 11803
(800) 537-2118
This free catalog includes daily living items such as grasp-able key holders, steady writing pens, easy-touch door handles, and more.

Maxi-Aids Aids and Appliances for the Blind, Visually Impaired, Physically Disabled, Hearing Impaired, and Senior Citizens with Special Needs
Maxi-Aids, Inc.
42 Executive Boulevard
P.O. Box 3209
Farmingdale, NY 11735
(800) 522-6294

References and Supporting Research

....

Bjorkman, D. J. "The Effect of Aspirin and Nonsteroidal Anti-Inflammatory Drugs on Prostaglandins." *American Journal of Medicine* 1998 Jul 27; 105(b):8S–12S.

Bolton, W. W. "Scientific Rationale for Specific Inhibition of COX-2." *Journal of Rheumatology Supplement* 1998 May; 51:2–7.

Cryer, B., et al. "Cyclooxygenase-1 and Cyclooxygenase-2 Selectivity of Widely Used Nonsteroidal Anti-Inflammatory Drugs." *American Journal of Medicine* 1998 May; 104(5):413–21.

"Detection of COX-1 and COX-2 Isoforms in Synovial Fluid Cells from Inflammatory Joint Diseases." *British Journal of Rheumatology* 1998 Jul; 37(7):733–8.

Dirig, D. M., et al. "Effect of COX-1 and COX-2 Inhibition on Induction and Maintenance of Carrageenan-Evoked Thermal Hyperalgesia in Rats." *Journal of Pharmacology Experimental Therapies* 1998 Jun; 285(3):1031–8.

Elder, D. J., et al. "COX-2 Inhibitors for Colorectal Cancer." *Nature Medicine* 1998 Apr; 4(4):392–3.

Fosslien, E. "Adverse Effects of Nonsteroidal Anti-Inflammatory Drugs on the Gastrointestinal System." *Annals of Clinical Laboratory Science* 1998 Mar–Apr; 28(2):67–81.

Kirsteins, A. E., Dietz, F., and Hwang, S. M. "Evaluating the Safety and Potential Use of a Weight-Bearing Exercise, Tai Chi Chuan, for Rheumatoid Arthritis Patients." *American Journal of Physical Medicine Rehabilitation* 1991 June; 70(3):136–141.

Lis-Balchin, M. "Essential Oils and 'Aromatherapy': Their Modern Role in Healing." *Journal of the Royal Society of Health* 1997 Oct; 117(5):324–9.

Lukiw, W. J., et al. "Budesonide Epimer R or Dexamethasone Selectively Inhibit Platelet-Activating Factor-Induced or Interleukin-1 Beta-Induced DNA Binding Activity of Cis-Acting Transcription Factors and Cyclooxygenase-2 Gene Expression in Human Epidermal Keratinocytes." *Proceedings of the National Academy of Sciences of the United States of America* 1998 Mar 31; 95(7):3914–9.

Schmassman, A. "Mechanisms of Ulcer Healing and Effects of Nonsteroidal Anti-Inflammatory Drugs." *American Journal of Medicine* 1998 Mar 30; 104(3A):43S–51S; discussion 79S–80S.

Seibert K., et al. "Distribution of COX-1 and COX-2 in Normal and Inflamed Tissues." *Advances in Experimental Medicine and Biology* 1997; 400A:167–70.

Simon, L. S. "Biology and Toxic Effects of Nonsteroidal Anti-Inflammatory Drugs." *Current Opinion in Rheumatology* 1998 May; 10(3):153–8.

Singer, I. I., et al. "Cyclooxygenase 2 Is Induced in Colonic Epithelial Cells in Inflammatory Bowel Disease." *Gastroenterology* 1998 Aug; 115(2):297–306.

Tsujii, M., et al. "Cyclooxygenase Regulates Angiogenesis Induced by Colon Cancer Cells." *Cell* 1998 May 29; 93(5):705–16.

Vane, J. R., et al. "Mechanism of Action of Anti-Inflammatory Drugs." *International Journal of Tissue Reactions* 1998; 20(1):3–15.

Vane, J. R., et al. "Cyclooxygenases 1 and 2." *Annual Review of Pharmacology Toxicology* 1998; 38:97–120.

Watson, A. J. "Chemopreventive Effects of NSAIDs Against Colorectal Cancer: Regulation of Apoptosis and Mitosis by COX-1 and COX-2." *Histology and Histopathology* 1998 Apr; 13(2):591–7.

Yeomans, N. D., et al. "Selective COX-2 Inhibitors: Are They Safe for the Stomach?" *Gastroenterology* 1998 Jul; 115(1):227–9

Glossary

....

A

Activities of daily living (ADLs). The activities we normally do in daily living, including feeding ourselves, bathing, dressing, grooming, work, homemaking, and leisure.

Acupuncture. The practice of putting needles into the body for health benefits, such as to reduce pain.

Aerobic exercise. Any exercise that promotes the oxygen circulation in the blood (running, cycling, swimming, and in-line skating).

Allergen. A substance such as pollen, mold, or animal dander that may produce an allergic reaction.

Alternative medicine. Healing therapies that are not usually scientific in nature or generally taught in medical schools.

ANAs. Antinuclear antibodies. ANAs are found in patients whose immune systems are prone to cause inflammation against their own body tissues. They are found in patients with a number of autoimmune diseases, such as systemic lupus erythematosus, Sjögren's syndrome, rheumatoid arthritis, polymyositis, and scleroderma.

Ankylosing spondylitis. A type of arthritis that causes chronic inflammation of the spine.

Antigen. Something potentially capable of inducing an immune response. Antigens elicit antibodies.

Anti-inflammatory. An agent that reduces inflammation without directly antagonizing the agent that caused it.

Apheresis. A technique in which blood is taken, treated or separated, then returned to the donor.

Arteritis, temporal. This serious inflammatory disease of the arteries is also called giant cell arteritis or cranial arteritis and is more common after age fifty. It is detected by a biopsy of an artery and is treated with cortisone. If left untreated, it can lead to blindness or stroke.

Arthritis. Inflammation of a joint that develops into swelling, stiffness, warmth, redness, and pain. There are more than one hundred types of arthritis, including osteoarthritis, rheumatoid arthritis, ankylosing spondylitis, psoriatic arthritis, lupus, gout, and pseudogout.

Arthritis, rheumatoid. An autoimmune disease characterized by chronic inflammation of the joints that can cause inflammation of tissues in other areas of the body (such as the lungs, heart, and eyes).

B

Back pain, low. Pain in the lower back that relates to the bony lumbar spine, discs between the vertebrae, ligaments around the spine and discs, spinal cord and nerves, muscles of the low back, internal organs of the pelvis and abdomen, and the skin covering the lumbar area.

Bone density test. A test for osteoporosis—thinning of the bones—which can lead to fractures and disability.

Bone scan. A test to identify abnormal areas of bone, stemming from problems such as fracture, infection, or cancer.

Bursitis. Inflammation of the bursa, a closed, fluid-filled sac that functions as a gliding surface to reduce friction between tissues of the body.

C

Calcium. A mineral in the body found mainly in the hard part of bones. Calcium is essential for healthy bones, as well as for muscle contraction, heart action, and normal blood clotting.

Food sources of calcium include dairy products, leafy green vegetables such as broccoli and collards, canned salmon, clams, oysters, calcium-fortified foods, and tofu.

Cartilage. Firm, rubbery tissue that cushions bones at joints.

Chronic. An illness or problem that lasts a long time, usually three months or more.

Clinical trials. Medical research studies conducted by government or private industry. Usually volunteers are recruited into "control groups" where experimental treatments for the detection, prevention, or cure of medical conditions are applied.

Corticosteroid. Any of the steroid hormones made by the cortex (outer layer) of the adrenal gland. Cortisol is a corticosteroid.

COX-1. One of two types of COX enzyme, it causes the production of the prostaglandins that help protect the stomach and other organs.

COX-2. The other type of COX enzyme, it causes the production of the prostaglandins that create inflammation and may be involved in some cancers, such as colon cancer, and in Alzheimer's disease.

D

Degenerative arthritis. *See* osteoarthritis.

Degenerative joint disease. *See* osteoarthritis.

F

Fibromyalgia. Also known as fibrositis or FMS (fibromyalgia syndrome), fibromyalgia causes chronic deep muscle pain, stiffness, and tenderness without detectable inflammation. Fibromyalgia does not cause body damage or deformity. However, undue fatigue plagues 90 percent of patients.

G

Gout. An arthritic condition characterized by abnormally elevated levels of uric acid in the blood, recurring attacks of joint inflammation (arthritis), deposits of hard lumps of uric acid in and around the joints, and decreased kidney function and kidney stones. The tendency to develop gout and elevated blood uric acid level (hyperuricemia) is often inherited and can be promoted by obesity, weight gain, alcohol intake, high blood pressure, abnormal kidney function, and drugs.

I

Inflammation. Localized redness, warmth, swelling, and pain because of infection, irritation, or injury.

Immune. Protected against infection.

Immune response. Any response by the immune system.

Internal medicine. A medical specialty dedicated to the diagnosis and medical treatment of adults. A physician who specializes in internal medicine is called an internist. A minimum of seven years of medical school and postgraduate training are focused on learning the prevention, diagnosis, and treatment of diseases of adults.

L

Lupus. *See* SLE.

N

NSAIDs (Nonsteroid anti-inflammatory drugs). Standard medications for the treatment of arthritis that help reduce inflammation and pain but may cause gastrointestinal upset.

Nodule. A small collection of tissue. The word *nodule* is the diminutive of *node* (a knot or knob) so a *nodule* means "a little knot or knob."

O

Orthopedics. The branch of surgery broadly concerned with the skeletal system (bones and joints).

Osteoarthritis. A type of arthritis caused by inflammation, breakdown, and eventual loss of the cartilage of the joints (also called degenerative arthritis or degenerative joint disease).

Osteoporosis. Thinning of the bones, with reduction in bone mass due to depletion of calcium and bone protein, predisposing to fractures.

Over-the-counter (OTC) drug. Drug for which a prescription is not needed.

P

Primary care. The "medical home" for a patient, ideally providing continuity and integration of health care. All family physicians and most pediatricians and internists are in primary care.

Prostaglandin. One of several types of proteins in the body, some of which are major contributors to inflammation and pain in arthritis, and others of which serve to protect the stomach and other organs.

Psoriatic arthritis. A potentially destructive and deforming form of arthritis that affects approximately 10 percent of persons with psoriasis.

R

Rheumatoid arthritis. An autoimmune disease, often called a "systemic" illness, which causes chronic inflammation of the joints and the tissue around the joints, as well as other organs in the body.

Rheumatoid factor. An antibody that is measurable in the blood. It is commonly used as a blood test for the diagnosis of rheumatoid arthritis. Rheumatoid factor is present in about 80 percent of adults (but a much lower proportion of children) with rheumatoid arthritis.

Rheumatoid nodules. Lumps that develop over joint areas that receive pressure, such as knuckles of the hand.

Rheumatologist. An internist who specializes in diseases of the bones, muscles, and joints.

S

Synovial fluid. The slippery fluid in joints.

Systemic lupus erythematosus (SLE). An inflammatory disease of connective tissue occurring predominantly in women (90 percent). It is considered an autoimmune disease.

T

Trigger points. Localized areas of tenderness around joints (not joints themselves) that hurt to touch.

Tumor necrosis factor (TNF). A protein produced in the body that is responsible for triggering inflammation in the joints, including pain, swelling, and probably also fatigue and joint destruction in rheumatoid arthritis.

About the Authors

....

Harris H. McIlwain, M.D., is board certified in rheumatology, internal medicine, and geriatric medicine. He is a graduate of Emory University Medical School and has practiced medicine with Tampa Medical Group for more than 20 years. *Town & Country* magazine recently named Dr. McIlwain one of the top 100 doctors in the United States. He is the coauthor of 13 books on aging, disease prevention, and pain relief.

Debra Fulghum Bruce is a Florida-based health journalist pursuing a doctorate in health communications. She has written more than 2,500 articles for women's and health magazines, such as *Woman's Day, Prevention,* and *Success.* She has also written 40 books on health and relationships and is the past editor of *Living Well Today,* a health/fitness/lifestyle publication.

Index

....